DESPERATION OF A DYING MAN

A Journey of Redemption and Healing

R. CORD BEATTY

Desperation Of A Dying Man

Copyright @ 2023 R. Cord Beatty
360 Media, LLC
R. Cord Beatty
368 East Riverside Drive #8
Saint George Utah, 84790

ISBN: 979-8-218-96080-3

All rights reserved. It is not legal to reproduce, duplicate, or transmit any part of this document in either electronic means or printed format. The recording of this publication is strictly prohibited.

TABLE OF CONTENTS

Chapter 1: Acknowledging the Void   1

Chapter 2: Understanding My Situation   45

Chapter 3: Exploring the Truth in Step One   67

Chapter 4: Confronting the Debts of Unmanageability   81

Chapter 5: Understanding Powerlessness. A Spiritual Journey   109

Chapter 6: Understanding the Power of Spiritual Surrender   123

Chapter 7: The Role of Ego in Powerlessness   133

Chapter 8: Spiritual Lessons from the Twelve Steps   151

Chapter 9: The Journey from Powerlessness to Empowerment   191

Chapter 10: Embracing the Power of Now   207

Chapter 11: Stories of Redemption   219

FOREWORD

In the ever-shifting tapestry of life, there comes a time for each of us when the wheels come off and we face the powerful convergence of adversity, spirituality, and self-discovery. For some, these struggles are compounded by mental illness or addiction. As an author immersed in this dynamic intersection, my intent for this foreword is to illuminate the concept of "hitting rock bottom," the understanding of powerlessness, and the profound surrender to a spiritual solution that marks the genesis of recovery and eventual freedom from suffering.

In the realm of mental illness and addiction, a common wisdom that echoes through the corridors of recovery is that profound understanding and experience with the first step of the Twelve-Step program can manifest a full recovery. This assertion, though initially skeptical, began to hold true in my life after a transformative encounter with step one, an encounter that was indeed a laborious journey through what I came to understand as "acceptable new lows."

The imagery of the 'bottom' in addiction and mental illness is a fluid one, often morphing through a sequence of progressively lower lows, each strangely acceptable until it no longer is. This may lead one to wonder: Do we ever find a 'true' bottom? Or is it just a continuous tumble down an endless chasm, ceaselessly seeking an acceptable low that remains elusive?

My own experiences narrate a tale of this tumultuous descent, marked by the wreckage of addiction and mental illness. Yet, it is not solely a story of pain and destruction. It is equally, if not more so, a story of spiritual awakening, redemption, and a journey to full recovery. Amid the ruins of my past life, once brimming with successful ventures in film and television, I found myself, at age forty-six, stripped of everything. My addiction and mental illness had claimed all; my marriage, children, business, home, money, and even my health.

My lowest point arrived in 2010, living homeless on the streets of Salt Lake City, where doctors predicted my imminent demise due to total liver failure and ensuing complications. However, at the precipice of death, standing amid the wreckage of my life, I experienced a spiritual awakening. I discovered, for the first time in my life, the power of God.

This awakening catalyzed a transformative journey that saw me not only recover from my alcoholism, addiction, and mental illness but also transform into a beacon of hope and support within the recovery community. With renewed purpose, I immersed myself in furthering my education, authoring books, founding treatment centers, and serving as a minister, public speaker, and mentor.

Despite my personal victories, I am acutely aware that each person stands at a unique juncture in their journey. You may be reading this at a point of desperate crossroads, akin to the desperation of a dying man, as I once was, or perhaps you are just beginning your journey toward the answers you need. Regardless, I invite you to approach the information in the pages of this book with an open mind and an open heart, casting aside the shroud of fear and prejudice that often accompanies the unknown.

This invitation isn't merely an exercise in futility. I promise, based on my own experience and the countless lives I've been privileged to help transform, that this information can serve as a catalyst for change. Embrace the prospect of a spiritual awakening, the concept of powerlessness, and the surrender to a spiritual solution. The journey may be arduous, marked by new lows and painful revelations, but the destination is one of full recovery, redemption, and, ultimately, freedom from suffering.

The purpose of this book and the words that follow is to be your beacon of hope, your guide as you navigate your personal journey in step one. It is my earnest desire to aid you in discovering your powerlessness over mental illness or addiction and guide you toward the transformative potential of surrendering to a spiritual solution.

This journey you're about to embark upon is about

finding your true power in what may initially seem like the most disempowering circumstances. In acknowledging your vulnerability and surrendering control, you carve a path for the higher powers to step in and light your way forward. In the middle of my darkest hour, lost on the fringes of society, alone and defeated, it was the light of spiritual awakening that guided me from the brink of death and despair. That light is available to everyone, even when we are mired in the depths of our personal "acceptable new lows."

But remember, this journey is not solely about reaching rock bottom, nor is it about the depth of the lows you endure. It's about recognizing when the "acceptable" has become "unacceptable," about gaining awareness of when it is time to reach upward instead of spiraling further downward. It's about choosing to rise from the ashes, spurred by the desperation of a dying man and the relentless determination of a phoenix ready to rise.

Indeed, the spiritual awakening, the psychic change that can lead to full recovery, doesn't transpire overnight. It's an ongoing journey that requires patience, perseverance, resilience, and, most importantly, an open heart. The book you're about to read isn't a quick fix, a magical cure-all. Instead, it's a compass guiding you through your spiritual voyage.

I stand today not as a symbol of perfection but as evidence of resilience and recovery. From living on the streets of Salt Lake City, grappling with mental illness and addiction, to pursuing a master's degree in psychology and addiction at Purdue University, becoming an author, a mentor, and the founder of recovery centers. I'm a testament to the transformative power of surrendering to a higher power, of embracing the spiritual solution.

So, as you turn the pages of your journey, I invite you to let go of the fear and skepticism. I encourage you to embrace the possibility of change. Be open to experiencing the profound power of the first step and the spiritual awakening that follows. Remember, there is a path to a cure, and it's a spiritual one, a journey toward freedom and a life beyond your current suffering. I invite you to step into this journey. As you do, remember this one promise: Step one has the power to change your life, just as it did mine.

CHAPTER 1

ACKNOWLEDGING THE VOID

Powerlessness is a term most associated with vulnerability, lack of control, and limitation, concepts that can stir unease in many individuals. Society often trains us to equate power with success, leading us to reject powerlessness. However, it is precisely this very notion of powerlessness that holds a transformative role in spiritual growth.

The term 'powerlessness' can evoke a sense of fear, discomfort, and perhaps even shame. It suggests a state of vulnerability, a lack of control, and limitations, which run counter to society's dominant narratives of success and achievement. Modern society idolizes power, whether it is financial, intellectual, physical, or social. It promotes the notion that to be successful, one must be powerful—capable of influencing circumstances and people around them, and in control of their own destiny.

However, the concept of powerlessness as it applies to spiritual growth is radically different from this societal norm. In the realm of spirituality, powerlessness does not mean weakness or failure. Instead, it represents a state of openness and humility that forms the foundation of deep personal and spiritual transformation.

When we accept our powerlessness, we come face to face with our own limitations and the hard truth that we can't control everything around us. This realization, while daunting, is also liberating. It invites us to let go of our attachments to outcomes, to our persistent need for control, and to our constant struggle against the current of life. It challenges the illusion of our ego, the constructed self-image that often drives us to seek control and deny our vulnerabilities.

This understanding is transformational because it shifts our perspective from resisting our reality to accepting and working within it. It teaches us that our strength lies not in rigid control but in our ability to adapt, accept, and flow with life's uncertainties.

In this sense, powerlessness becomes a gateway to profound spiritual growth. It opens the door to surrender, acceptance, and, ultimately, a deeper connection with the universal forces that guide our lives. This is a radical shift in perspective that moves us away from fear and resistance, toward love, acceptance, and harmony with the natural order of life. So, rather than a weakness, powerlessness becomes a path to profound strength, resilience, and wisdom.

The Dao De Jing, written by the ancient Chinese philosopher Lao Tzu, promotes a worldview that encourages harmonious living with nature and oneself, embracing the inherent balance and flow of life, often referred to as the Dao or Tao. The philosophy underscores the principle of "Wu Wei," or "effortless action," a state of being where one acts in alignment with the Dao, suggesting that we are most effective when we surrender our personal will to the natural course of life. This surrendering isn't about capitulation or defeat but an acknowledgment of the natural flow of life's events, which are often outside of our control.

The first step of the Twelve Steps of AA echoes the wisdom of the Dao in many ways. It guides us to embark on a transformative journey by acknowledging the reality of addiction effortlessly. Surrendering to this truth is not a defeat or resignation but a courageous acceptance of what is—a recognition of the natural currents of life, often beyond our control. It is an act of empowerment, releasing the illusion of control and embracing the path of recovery.

In this surrender, we open ourselves to the profound forces of a higher power, just as aligning with the Dao connects us to the invisible guiding hand of the universe. Instead of struggling against the world, we learn to flow with it, finding our true potential and unlocking the power within. It is through this alignment that we discover peace, purpose, and the ability to navigate life's challenges with grace and ease.

When I took my first step on the path of recovery, it felt as if I had stepped into a vast ocean of wisdom, an endless wellspring of insights that spoke to the depths of my being. Among those insights, the Dao stood as a pillar of guidance, a steadfast companion on my journey.

The Dao was not a distant concept to me; it was a palpable presence, permeating every aspect of my existence. I witnessed its essence in the changing seasons, in the symphony of nature, and in the beating of my heart. It was the subtle force that orchestrated the dance of life, a cosmic conductor leading the rhythm of the universe.

What enchanted me most about the Dao was its gentle nature, its ability to guide without force. It wasn't a rigid path to follow but a harmonious flow to embrace. It did not demand control but invited surrender. It was a melody I could only hear when I quieted the noise of my own desires and listened to the symphony of existence.

And so, I discovered that living in harmony with the Dao meant relinquishing the need to struggle and instead surrender to life's currents. It was a dance of adaptation, a journey of fluidity. Like a river, I learned to navigate obstacles with resilience and power, yet never losing my softness. By embracing the Dao wisdom, I learned the art of dancing with life, stepping lightly yet purposefully, and finding my way with grace.

In the union of the first step of the Twelve Steps and the wisdom of the Dao, I found liberation from the chains of addiction and a path to authentic living. Both teach us that surrender is not a defeat but a gateway to freedom. By humbly accepting our limitations, acknowledging the forces beyond our control, and aligning ourselves with a higher power or the universal flow, we discover the strength to transcend our challenges and embrace the fullness of life.

> *"We admitted we were powerless over alcohol—that our lives had become unmanageable."*

The implicit acknowledgement of powerlessness is a crucial first step toward recovery. It's an admission of the limits of personal willpower in overcoming addiction. By accepting our inability to control the addiction, we surrender to a higher power that can provide strength and guidance.

Alcoholics Anonymous (AA), a fellowship aimed at helping individuals recover from alcoholism, is based on a twelve-step program of spiritual and character development. The first of these steps states, "We admitted we were powerless over alcohol—that our lives had become unmanageable." This admission is the bedrock upon which the entire program is built.

The idea of powerlessness in this context may seem counterintuitive at first, especially when we are taught to believe in the power of personal will and determination. However, in the realm of addiction, admitting powerlessness is crucial. It signifies the acknowledgment that alcoholism is a disease that one cannot conquer through willpower alone.

This admission is twofold: Firstly, it requires the recognition of one's addictions or mental illness, a step that can be challenging for many, as it involves coming face-to-face with a harsh reality that one might have been denying or avoiding. Secondly, it necessitates the acceptance of the fact that the addiction has made life unmanageable, that it is beyond one's control to rectify the situation without help.

This is where the concept of surrender becomes central. By accepting powerlessness over the addiction, the individual can then surrender the struggle to a higher power. The higher power concept doesn't have to be religious or even spiritual; it simply represents anything greater than oneself that can offer strength, guidance, and support. For some, this may be God, while for others, it may be the collective wisdom of the AA group.

This surrender is not a sign of weakness or failure; rather, it's a courageous act of honesty, humility, and openness. It's the recognition that one needs help, which, in turn, creates the necessary space for that help to enter. It's the starting point of a journey that can lead to recovery and personal transformation.

In admitting powerlessness and surrendering to a higher power, we began to relinquish the ego, pride, and stubborn self-will that often fuel addiction. We start to open ourselves up to the possibility of change and healing. We take the first critical step on the path to recovery, a path that leads away from the isolation of addiction and toward the promise of a healthier, more balanced life.

My struggle with alcohol was a battle I fought in the deepest trenches of my soul. I pored over the Big Book of Alcoholics Anonymous and studied its teachings, looking for a hint, a key to unraveling this tight knot of desperation.

As I skimmed through page twenty of the book, it gently nudged me toward a realization. It was a beacon that signaled the beginning of my journey toward recovery: the twelve-step journey, starting with the crucial first one. "We admitted we 'were' powerless over alcohol and that our lives have become unmanageable." It was a vivid moment. An opening of my eyes and inner release.

But let me tell you, it wasn't as simple as just declaring I'm an alcoholic. I found that this popular notion was a delusion. The idea that admitting you're an alcoholic at a meeting or a treatment program is enough is just a myth.

The Big Book, on page thirty, emphasizes that the first step toward full recovery is truly conceding to your innermost self that you "were" alcoholic, breaking free from the delusion that we are like others. It is written in past tense. This understanding is essential, yet it's often misconstrued. There's a mistaken belief that the twelve steps are just "suggestions," but that's far from the truth. Calling myself an alcoholic is one thing, but what truly defines me as someone suffering from this disease? What aspects of my experiences make it undeniable? There are countless people who refer to themselves as alcoholics because they attend AA meetings, undergo treatments, or simply because they drink excessively. They often talk about addictive behaviors, cravings, and loss of control but fail to comprehend the essence of their struggle with alcoholism.

You must ask yourself hard questions about your personal journey. How can I accept my condition if I don't fully comprehend what it means to be an alcoholic/addict? Just admitting, accepting, and surrendering isn't enough. It's a fundamental misunderstanding of the first step. The key to recovery lies in fully conceding to my innermost self that I have a disease—whether that's alcoholism, addiction, or mental illness—before I can truly admit, accept, and surrender to it.

This struggle reminded me of a frustrating cycle. Each failed attempt at sobriety was followed by a brief period of relief, only to relapse again and again. This repetitive cycle was my worst enemy; I was trapped within my own struggle with alcohol, like a hamster in a wheel, running relentlessly but getting nowhere.

The first step, as defined by Alcoholics Anonymous, is to admit powerlessness over alcohol, but that seemed vague and elusive to me. What does it even mean? What does it mean to be powerless? The understanding came gradually as I sought to answer this question, and it changed my perspective significantly.

My problem with alcohol wasn't just about losing control over my drinking. Alcohol had a much more profound effect on me: it transformed my perception of reality. The minute alcohol trickled down my throat, it painted a distorted picture of the world around me. I loved this deception. I could escape from the 'duck' I was and soar high like an eagle. This escape was what I had unknowingly obsessed about.

However, the more I drank, the less effective this escape became. I found myself drinking yet still feeling like a duck, no matter how hard I tried to fly like an eagle. I continued drinking until it started causing serious consequences, like loss of career, marriage, home, hospitalization, and legal trouble. I found myself drinking not because I wanted the effects but to satisfy an insatiable obsession of my mind that had trapped me in an unending cycle. Sound familiar?

This uncontrolled drinking, the obsession, and the consequent physical craving for more alcohol was what differentiated me from others, what made me an alcoholic. And no one can become an alcoholic if they do not have the genetic disposition to addiction. That would be impossible.

One day, during a time of homelessness and desperation, I found myself in a cheap motel, staring at my reflection in the cracked bathroom mirror, my face washed pale by the cold fluorescent light. I glanced at my once jovial eyes that now looked back with a tiredness that couldn't be masked. No laughter, no warmth. Just the dull gaze of a person who had lost his battle with the bottle. Someone who was hopelessly defeated.

It wasn't like I hadn't tried to get out of its grasp. Countless mornings spent promising myself to never touch the devil's juice again, never-ending meetings, stints of sobriety, multiple treatment centers, counselors, and therapists, only to find myself uncorking another bottle once again. This routine was as predictable as the changing seasons.

I had visited a string of AA meetings, where everyone would embrace newcomers with open arms, letting them know they weren't alone. I admired their strength, their resilience, their progress. And even though they would always remind me, 'Admitting you're an alcoholic is the first step,' somehow, it just didn't resonate with me.

So, I would nod, agree, and even raise my hand to admit my struggle. But it didn't change anything. I was still in the same dark place. It was like trying to fix a gaping wound with a Band-Aid. Sure, it might look like you're doing something, but the injury is still there, festering underneath.

One day, after another trip to the ER that almost killed me, I found myself flipping through the Big Book once again, looking for answers. I read and reread the steps, and suddenly, the first one hit me in a different way. I read something that I had not noticed before. It was not about saying that I'm an alcoholic. It was about acknowledging the grip alcohol had over me and how it had turned my life upside down.

Suddenly, I felt an icy shiver go down my spine, making me sit upright. I finally *understood*. It was about fully conceding to myself that I was indeed suffering from this disease. It wasn't enough to just say it out loud in a room full of people, I had to truly believe it, feel it in the depths of my soul. It wasn't about surrender but about complete acceptance.

I realized, to admit, accept, and surrender to my condition, I had to first concede to my deepest self that I had the disease of addiction. Only then could I embark on the journey to recovery. It was a profound moment. The struggle that seemed so complex was suddenly distilled into a simple truth. It was like a light breaking through the darkness.

Alcohol had turned my world upside down, and I realized that it didn't just distort my perception, it fundamentally altered who I was. I wasn't living my life; I was a puppet being controlled by my addiction. This realization was as shocking as it was liberating.

But the real battle had just begun. I knew this new revelation wasn't going to be a magic cure. There were going to be setbacks, relapses, times when I would find myself at the bottom of the pit again. But this time, I was equipped with a deeper understanding of my disease.

I recognized the cycle, the obsession, the craving, the loss of control. And although I knew it was going to be a long and arduous journey, for the first time, I felt a flicker of hope.

For years, alcohol had altered my reality, making me believe I was soaring when I was in fact sinking. But now, even though I was at the lowest point in my life, I felt grounded. It was a strange, paradoxical feeling.

I knew then that admitting my powerlessness wasn't about confessing my weakness. Instead, it was about accepting the gravity of my situation. It was the first brick in the foundation of my recovery. I had a disease, a disease that had been insidiously gnawing at me from the inside out, but in that moment, I felt its grip on me start to loosen. It was as if I had taken the first step out of a dark tunnel into the light.

I wasn't naive, though. I knew that acknowledging the problem was just the beginning of a long, uphill battle, a journey filled with trials and tribulations. But I was ready. Or at least, I believed I was more prepared than I had ever been before. This newfound realization had finally shown me a clear path to a connection with a higher power. Steps two and three took on new meaning for me. I had a transformed connection with a God of my understanding and could accept it.

The next AA meeting I attended took on a whole new

meaning for me. I wasn't there to passively listen to others' stories or to mechanically repeat the words that were expected of me. I was there to heal. I shared my realization with the group, my voice trembling with the gravity of my words. There was an uncomfortable silence as I bared my soul, but it was followed by an outpouring of support and understanding. I wasn't alone in my battle; these people were my allies. I was no longer homeless.

And so, my journey to recovery began. Each day was a battle, a fight against my inner demons. But with each passing day, the obsessions grew a bit weaker, the need a bit less urgent. My commitment to prayer and meditation became stronger. There were moments of weakness, of course, moments when the bottle seemed like an old friend calling me back. But I held on. Days turned into weeks and weeks into months. I became stronger and stronger with each passing day.

I kept track of my progress, marking each sober day with a triumphant tick on my calendar. Every tick was a victory, a symbol of my strength and resilience and a reprieve from my addiction through God's grace.

Despite my progress, the fear of relapse always lingered in the back of my mind. I knew that recovery wasn't a linear path, that there would be bumps and detours along the way. And indeed, there were moments when I stumbled and fell. But with each fall, I learned to get back up stronger, more determined and more spiritually connected.

The turning point came after a year of sobriety. I had finished my work in the twelve steps and had gained the promises held within. I found myself at a social gathering, surrounded by laughter, music, and flowing alcohol. There was a time when I couldn't imagine being in such a setting without a drink in my hand. But that night, as I clutched my glass of sparkling water, I realized that I didn't need alcohol to be sociable, to laugh, to enjoy life.

That night, I went home and looked at myself in the mirror, a ritual I had avoided for so long. But this time, the face looking back at me was different. The eyes were still tired, but there was a spark in them, a spark of hope and determination for my new life.

My battle with alcoholism was far from over, but I had come a long way. Admitting my powerlessness over alcohol was the first step, but each step that followed was equally crucial. Each step brought me closer to reclaiming my life, my identity.

Interestingly, the teachings of Lao Tzu and the philosophy of AA intersect at the point of surrender. Both imply that there is a 'higher power' at work, whether it is the natural course of the universe or a spiritual entity acknowledged in AA. By surrendering control to this higher power, we can align ourselves with life's flow, providing space for change, growth, and recovery.

In both contexts, acknowledging our limitations and powerlessness is the beginning of transformation. It is about accepting the truth of our human condition, our fragility, and the fact that there are things in life that we cannot change or control. This acceptance doesn't diminish us but instead opens us up to new possibilities and the potential for spiritual growth. By embracing our powerlessness, we let go of the futile struggle against life's currents and instead learn to flow with them, ultimately creating space for healing and self-transformation. It is a cornerstone of wisdom in both spiritual teachings and steps toward recovery.

This alignment of wisdom across the Daoist philosophy and the AA approach provides a deeper, more nuanced understanding of the human condition and the journey toward personal transformation and spiritual growth. Embracing our powerlessness, acknowledging our limitations, and surrendering to a higher power are common threads that weave through both philosophies.

It is through this surrender, this letting go of control, that we open ourselves up to experience life in a fuller, more authentic way. The illusion of control often creates a barrier between us and our experiences, leading us to resist or deny the realities of life. But when we acknowledge our powerlessness and accept the truth of our limitations, we break down this barrier, allowing life to flow freely through us.

In this state of surrender, we become more receptive to life's teachings, more attuned to its rhythms, and more able to respond to its challenges with wisdom and grace. We start to see that our struggles and challenges aren't obstacles to our growth but rather opportunities for learning and transformation. This shift in perspective can have a profound effect on our lives, opening us up to newfound peace, resilience, and personal growth.

Surrendering to a higher power doesn't mean giving up our agency or responsibility. Instead, it enables us to harness the power of these greater forces in our journey toward transformation. By aligning ourselves with the wisdom of the higher power, we become active participants in our own healing and growth.

Embracing powerlessness and surrendering to a higher power is not a sign of defeat but a courageous step toward freedom. It marks the beginning of a journey—a journey from denial and resistance to acceptance and alignment, from struggle and suffering to healing and growth, from isolation and despair to community and hope. Whether it's aligning with the Dao, walking the path of recovery in AA, or just living life committed to daily prayer and meditation, this journey is ultimately about returning to our true selves, finding our place in the world, and living in harmony with life's ebb and flow.

To fully understand and have a profound first step experience, we must understand what we are dealing with. Alcoholism and addiction are diseases like cancer, multiple sclerosis, diabetes, or heart disease. Addition has two parts to the disease. An allergy of my body and an obsession of my mind, which make it different than other diseases. Because of the differences, it needs to be treated differently. And there is no magic pill. An individual who is suffering from the disease has to work hard for a positive outcome.

Dr. Silkworth's understanding of alcoholism found in the book of Alcoholics Anonymous plays a significant role in the interpretation of the first of the Twelve Steps: "We admitted we were powerless over alcohol—that our lives had become unmanageable."

He introduces the idea of alcoholism as a physical issue, not a mental one, stemming from a phenomenon he terms the 'phenomenon of craving.' This phenomenon refers to the uncontrollable desire that takes over an alcoholic after taking the first drink of the day. According to Dr. Silkworth, this craving is so overpowering that nothing else matters—not important meetings, not responsibilities, not the potential negative consequences. It's as if all the world shrinks down to the singular need for more alcohol.

The key point here is that the craving isn't a result of lack of willpower or moral strength. It is a physical response akin to an allergic reaction, an abnormal reaction to alcohol that only occurs after the substance has been introduced into the body. This is crucial in understanding powerlessness over alcohol—it's not about being weak or flawed, it's about the body reacting to a substance in a way that we can't control.

In the book of Alcoholics Anonymous, where the first step is found, forty-three pages are devoted just to step one. On page xxviii, paragraph one, one of the authors, Dr. Silkworth, discusses his belief that alcohol's effect on chronic alcoholics is a manifestation of an allergy. This perspective reframes the way we understand alcoholism. If we consider alcoholism as an allergy—an abnormal physiological response to a substance—then it becomes clear that the individual suffering from this allergy is powerless over their reaction to alcohol.

This brings new weight to the first step of the Twelve Steps. Acknowledging that we are dealing with a physical, allergic reaction rather than a moral failing or a lack of willpower can make the admission of powerlessness less of a blow to our self-esteem and more of a scientific understanding of our body's response. It is a compassionate perspective that paves the way for accepting our powerlessness and seeking help.

Ultimately, this understanding of alcoholism doesn't absolve us of responsibility for our recovery. Instead, it helps us to see more clearly what we're up against and underscores the importance of avoiding that first drink—the one that triggers the phenomenon of craving. This physical understanding complements the psychological and spiritual journey of the Twelve Steps, providing a comprehensive approach to recovery.

As we embrace the wisdom of the first step, we realize that powerlessness isn't about defeat. On the contrary, it's about acknowledging the nature of our condition. The confession of powerlessness over alcohol is the first step toward empowering ourselves to make changes that lead to recovery.

It's important to note that while we admit powerlessness over the physical craving for alcohol, we are not powerless over our actions. We still retain the authority of choice. We may not be able to control our body's reaction to alcohol, but we can choose whether we take that first drink. This is where our true power lies—in the decision to abstain from the substance that triggers our craving.

In a way, understanding alcoholism as an allergy aid's in recognizing the necessity of step one. It would be irrational to blame oneself for sneezing when exposed to pollen, right? Likewise, it becomes illogical to fault oneself for experiencing the physical craving associated with the consumption of alcohol. As such, accepting powerlessness becomes less about admitting defeat and more about understanding the facts of one's condition.

What Dr. Silkworth's work does is lend scientific validity to the principles embodied in the Twelve Steps. By explaining that the 'phenomenon of craving' is a physical reaction, much like an allergy, he provides a concrete, biological explanation for why the first drink sets off a chain reaction for an alcoholic. He reinforces the idea that our fight isn't against our willpower or moral strength but against an abnormal physiological response.

In essence, we admit that we are powerless over alcohol—that our lives had become unmanageable, but we do so armed with the knowledge of why this is so. And with that comprehension, we reclaim our power, because hadn't been able to pinpoint the root of our problem and, more importantly, find the solution. We recognize our inability to moderate our drinking once we've started but also realize our capability to choose not to start at all.

The acknowledgment of our powerlessness, therefore, becomes our strongest asset. It propels us into the following steps with honesty, openness, and a clear understanding of the enemy we're up against, preparing us for the transformative journey ahead.

Admitting powerlessness over alcohol—the fact that our lives had become unmanageable—forces us to confront our vulnerability, but also invites us to make a shift in perception. This shift is crucial for recovery. It brings a change to our way of thinking and reshapes our understanding of control.

Previously, we might have tried to exert control over our drinking, attempting to limit our intake, determine what we drank, or set boundaries on when and where we drank. Such efforts often proved fruitless, further proving our powerlessness over the substance. However, by admitting this powerlessness, we come to understand that our control shouldn't be focused on trying to moderate the drinking. Instead, our control should be centered on the decision not to drink at all.

Through admitting our powerlessness, we clear the path to take control over what truly is within our grasp. It's not about gaining control over the alcohol or the craving; it's about gaining control over ourselves and our actions.

This is where the paradox of powerlessness reaches its crescendo—the confession of our weakness becomes our strength. The realization of our inability to control our drinking is the key to taking control of our lives.

Furthermore, Dr. Silkworth's comparison of alcoholism to an allergy adds a physical, tangible facet to the understanding of this first step. It provides a concrete reason for why we cannot control our reaction once we start drinking. It's not a moral failing or a lack of willpower—it's a physiological response. And it's one that we can choose not to activate.

This realization becomes our steppingstone, a foundation to recovery. As we proceed with the remaining steps, this awareness remains with us. It teaches us humility, brings clarity, and guides us on our journey. From here, we start reconstructing our lives, not as victims of an uncontrollable craving but as empowered individuals who have chosen to reclaim control over our lives. The paradox of powerlessness is that it becomes the foundation upon which we build our newfound strength and freedom.

The journey from powerlessness to empowerment doesn't end with merely acknowledging the problem and understanding the physiological aspect of alcoholism. It goes deeper than that. It involves the continuous process of cultivating self-awareness, developing emotional resilience, and fostering a commitment to personal growth and change. And this entire process begins with an admission of powerlessness—a paradox that turns our perceived weakness into an opportunity for transformation.

After we come to terms with the fact that we have no control over our craving once alcohol is in our system, we begin to foster a sense of responsibility toward our wellbeing. This, in essence, becomes a practice of empowerment—a conscious choice to refrain from the one act that sparks the allergic reaction. It's not about managing the craving after it has started but about preempting the craving altogether. We learn to leverage our power in the best possible way, by controlling our actions and deciding not to drink.

Additionally, when we admit our powerlessness, we also open ourselves up to receive help and support from others. The notion of 'going it alone' is shed. The acceptance of our condition encourages us to seek help from a higher power, from our peers, from medical professionals, and from the broader community. We begin to realize that although we are powerless over alcohol, we are not powerless over our lives. In fact, we gain strength and power through our shared experiences, communal support, and combined knowledge. We are empowered by the very act of surrendering, accepting, and reaching out.

Through this lens, the first step in the Twelve Steps, "We admitted we were powerless over alcohol—that our lives had become unmanageable," not only paves the way for recovery but also serves as a guide for a new way of life. It reminds us that we are not defined by our past mistakes or our physical predispositions. Instead, we are defined by our resilience, our ability to change, and our determination to take control of our lives, regardless of the challenges we face. This is the power of paradox, the paradox of powerlessness: it is the doorway to a journey of self-discovery, transformation, and ultimate empowerment.

Acknowledging our powerlessness, we lay down the weight of our past struggles. We break free from the cycle of repeated failures and disappointments. We start to realize that our past does not have to define our future. We are not doomed to repeat our past mistakes. We are not destined to live an unmanageable life. We have the power to rewrite our story.

As we go through the subsequent steps of the program, we learn to trust ourselves, to forgive ourselves, and to love ourselves. We discover that we can make healthy decisions and establish a fulfilling life. We uncover our inner strength and resilience, and we build up our capacity to handle life's ups and downs without resorting to alcohol.

Admitting our powerlessness is not a sign of weakness but a recognition of our condition and a pivotal moment of courage. It is a radical act of honesty, humility, and bravery. It's the moment we stop running from our problems and start facing them head-on. It's the moment we decide to take back control of our lives. By embracing our powerlessness, we become more powerful than we ever thought possible.

This is the transformative power of the first step. It's a powerful reminder that change starts with us and that no matter how difficult or impossible our situation may seem, we always have the power to choose a different path. We always have the power to change. This is the paradox of powerlessness, the paradox that makes recovery possible.

When Dr. Bob labeled alcoholism as an allergy, he used a medical term to describe a condition that is unique to those suffering from this illness. Much like a person with a shellfish allergy who experiences physical discomfort and potentially dangerous reactions upon consumption, an alcoholic experiences an abnormal, almost allergic, reaction to alcohol. However, unlike a typical allergy, the reaction here is not hives or difficulty breathing but an overwhelming craving that makes moderation and control virtually impossible.

What my mentors wanted me to realize through asking these questions was the extent to which my life was being impacted by alcohol. Did I have an abnormal reaction to alcohol when I drank it? Yes. Upon consuming that first drink, all bets were off. A switch would flip, the craving would take over, and no matter how much I drank, it was never enough.

Did I understand what he meant by 'abnormal'? Initially, I didn't. What was abnormal about wanting to let loose, have fun, and forget about my problems? But as he explained further, it started to make sense. He was referring to the chaos, the confusion, and the memory blackouts that were my constant companions. The loss of control that ensued after the first sip, leading to behavior that was reckless, dangerous, and completely out of character. The kind of behavior that a normal drinker would seldom, if ever, engage in.

The two a.m. drunken calls and the subsequent confused conversations were all too familiar. They were a perfect illustration of the abnormality he was talking about. While under the influence of alcohol, I would often make promises, commitments, and confessions that I had no recollection of the next morning. The alcohol-induced amnesia would leave me scrambling to piece together the fragments of my conversations and actions.

And the mornings after? The guilt, the confusion, the frantic attempts to remember and mend the damage done the previous night? Those were all signs of an abnormal reaction to alcohol. They were manifestations of the allergy that Dr. Bob spoke about.

I started to see my drinking in a new light. I recognized that I was allergic to alcohol in the sense that I had an abnormal reaction to it. This realization was both terrifying and liberating. Terrifying because I finally acknowledged the magnitude of my problem and liberating because I now had a better understanding of why I behaved the way I did when I drank. It wasn't a lack of willpower or moral failing but an allergic reaction to alcohol that led to my powerlessness and unmanageable life. This realization marked the beginning of my journey to recovery. It was the first step toward acknowledging my powerlessness and starting to make changes.

Every person who suffers from mental illness or addiction and has fully recovered has the same story of recovery. The circumstances may be different, but the journey and the outcome are generally the same. Why? Because someone suffering from addiction or mental illness must first gain a deep desire to change. We must be willing participants in the recovery process. There is no therapist, psychiatrist, counselor, magic potion, lotion, or pill that can cure addiction or mental illness. It takes a mental change that is brought on through a spiritual awakening. For this to happen, one has to be willing to participate and to do hard work to get it.

Every story of recovery from mental illness or addiction indeed shares a common thread—a profound, personal transformation often referred to as a "spiritual awakening." However, this doesn't necessarily mean a religious experience but rather an awakening to a new way of thinking, feeling, and interacting with the world. It signifies an internal shift, a change of perspective, an enlightened understanding of oneself and one's place in the world.

Whether it's battling alcoholism, drug addiction, depression, anxiety, or any other mental illness, the journey toward recovery begins with an individual's deep desire to change. It's an acknowledgment of the problem and a willingness to seek and accept help. It's about recognizing that they're not alone in their struggles and that it's okay to ask for assistance. But most importantly, it's about developing the willingness to do the hard work that recovery entails.

Because recovery is indeed hard work. It requires the courage to face one's fears and traumas, the strength to confront and overcome one's negative patterns of thinking and behavior, the patience to learn new coping skills and strategies, and the persistence to keep going even when progress seems slow or nonexistent.

No therapist, psychiatrist, counselor, or medication can do this work for an individual. They can provide guidance, support, tools, and strategies, but ultimately, it's up to the individual to put these into practice and to effect the necessary changes in their life. This is why participation and hard work are so crucial in the recovery process.

This doesn't mean that medication or therapy aren't essential components of the treatment plan. They often are. But they're tools, not cures. They can help manage symptoms, provide insights, and facilitate change, but they can't force it.

Real, lasting change comes from within. It's brought about by a mental change, a radical shift in one's mindset and outlook. It's about developing a new understanding of oneself and one's illness, a new way of relating to oneself and the world. It's about adopting healthier habits, attitudes, and coping strategies. It's about growing, evolving, and becoming a better version of oneself.

And this transformation doesn't happen overnight. It's a journey, a process, often a long and difficult one. But it's also a journey of self-discovery, growth, and empowerment. It's a voyage that ultimately leads to a healthier, happier, more fulfilling life. This is the common thread that runs through every story of recovery from mental illness or addiction. This is the shared journey, the shared outcome. Because at the end of the day, recovery isn't about getting back to where one was before the illness, it's about moving forward to a better, healthier place.

But how do we get there? How do we move from a place of suffering to a place of recovery? It starts, as I've said before, with the deep desire to change. But desire alone isn't enough. We also need faith—faith in ourselves, faith in the process, faith in the possibility of a better future.

We need to believe that change is possible, that recovery is possible, and that we have the power within ourselves to make it happen.

Then, we must commit to doing the work, to actively participating in the recovery process. We must show up for therapy, meetings, treatment, practice our coping strategies, and actively work on changing our thought and behavior patterns. We must take responsibility for our recovery and for making the changes we want to see in our lives.

And it won't be easy. There will be setbacks, struggles, and moments of doubt. There may be times when we question whether recovery is even possible. But it's in these moments that we must remind ourselves of why we started this journey in the first place. We must remind ourselves of our desire to change, our faith in recovery, and our commitment to doing the work.

One of the most important things we can do in these moments is to reach out to others—our therapist, our support group, our loved ones. They can provide us with the encouragement, support, and perspective we need to keep going. They can remind us of how far we've come and how much we've achieved. And they can reassure us that recovery is indeed possible, even when it doesn't feel like it.

But perhaps the most important part of the recovery process is learning to love and accept ourselves. This means accepting our past, our mistakes, our struggles, and our illness. It means acknowledging that these are part of who we are but they don't define us. We are more than our illness, more than our past. We are individuals with strengths, talents, dreams, and potential. We are deserving of love, respect, and happiness.

Taking a deep breath, I asked myself, "Do I have the power to simply change my perspective on alcohol and drinking without any assistance?" In all honesty, if I could magically alter my thinking and behavior, wouldn't I have done it already? Why would I need the Twelve Steps, AA, or a sponsor? Why not just stop drinking?

There's a difficult truth here. Changing lifelong habits and deeply ingrained thought patterns is not easy, and rarely is it something we can do on our own. I know this from my own experience. If I could have changed on my own, I would have. But I couldn't, and that's why I needed help.

The next question is even harder. Am I willing to undergo a complete psychic change? Am I ready to let go of my old self, my old ways, and become something new? This isn't a small tweak or a minor adjustment. This is a fundamental, ground-up transformation of who I am and how I perceive the world.

According to Dr. Silkworth's opinion found in the book of Alcoholics Anonymous, on page xxix, such a psychic change requires something beyond human power. This aligns with the authors' suggestion that without a complete psychic change, there is little hope for recovery. And crucially, they stress that this change cannot come from a human source.

Pause to let that sink in. Can a sponsor or a spouse cause this psychic change in me? Can my children? Can worldly possessions like money, house, car, boat, or clothes bring about this transformation? They all play important roles in my life, and they all influence me in various ways. But can they instigate the profound change that I need to recover from my addiction?

The text suggests that they can't. It implies that something more, something beyond human understanding and power, is needed to produce this essential psychic change. And this, it says, is the key to recovery.

So, I have to ask myself again: Am I willing to accept this? Am I willing to admit that I need help from a higher power, that I can't do this on my own? Am I willing to embrace the possibility of a complete mental change? The question hangs in the air, waiting for an answer. I take another deep breath, ready to face the truth of my situation. As uncomfortable as it may be, it's a necessary step on the path to recovery.

As I continue to reflect on this idea, I remember how terrifying the thought of change was when I first came into the rooms of AA. I was resistant, because change, even change for the better, often involves a loss of what's familiar. I had built an identity around alcohol, it was my comfort, my solace, and my go-to solution for everything. Giving it up meant venturing into uncharted territory.

But as I sit here, years into my journey of sobriety, I realize how important the acceptance of powerlessness and the willingness for a mental change were for my recovery. They were the foundation, the cornerstones upon which the rest of my recovery was built. And while I initially thought of them as an admission of defeat, I now see them as a declaration of hope.

In embracing my powerlessness, I learned that surrender wasn't about giving up but about being open to receiving help, guidance, and strength from a power greater than myself. In being open to a cognitive change, I gave myself permission to let go of destructive thought patterns and behaviors and to allow something new to take their place.

I've come to understand that neither my mentor, my spouse, my children, nor any material possessions could bring about the internal shift required for my recovery. They were, and continue to be, vital support, sources of love, motivation, and assistance, but the change, the profound transformation of my inner self, had to come from a higher power and my willingness to allow it to work within me.

I've discovered that recovery isn't about reaching a destination but about embracing a continuous journey of growth and transformation. It's about learning to live one day at a time, facing whatever comes my way with courage and faith in a power greater than myself. And it all starts with admitting my powerlessness and being open to inner renovation.

As I consider this, I find myself filled with gratitude for my journey, the good and the bad. For the pain that brought me to my knees and for the power that lifted me up. For the transformation that has allowed me to live a life of purpose and sobriety, and for the continuing journey, always reminding me to remain humble, open, and willing to grow.

I ask myself once more, am I willing to continue? Am I willing to embrace change, even when it's uncomfortable, even when it's challenging? And I find, with quiet certainty, the answer is yes. Always yes. Because this journey, though challenging, has given me a life beyond my wildest dreams. A life not defined by alcohol but by freedom, growth, and a sense of peace that comes from living in harmony with a power greater than myself.

Indeed, the journey to sobriety, the journey toward an intimate, mental shift, is not a solitary endeavor. As I delve deeper into this process, I find that it involves building a new relationship, not just with myself but also with a power greater than myself.

The beauty of the Twelve Steps and organizations like Alcoholics Anonymous and other such programs is that they provide a community of individuals who are on a similar path. They provide a space where we can share our struggles and triumphs, learn from each other's experiences, and find solace in the knowledge that we are not alone. And they provide a sponsor who guides us through the steps, not as a superior but as a fellow traveler who has walked the path before us.

Despite this communal aspect, the journey is still profoundly personal. After all, no one else can admit my powerlessness for me. No one else can undergo the mental change on my behalf. These are things that I, and I alone, must do. However, knowing that there are others who have done so, who have faced the same fears and overcome the same obstacles, provides a source of strength and inspiration.

Admitting powerlessness over alcohol, surrendering to a higher power, and undergoing a psychic change are not passive acts. They require active participation, a deliberate choice to let go of old habits, to challenge old beliefs, and to open oneself to new ways of thinking and being. They require courage, patience, and an unwavering commitment to the journey.

As I move forward, I constantly ask myself, am I willing to remain open to the possibility of change? Am I willing to keep learning, keep growing, keep evolving? I know now that recovery is not a destination but an ongoing process, a constant unfolding of the self in relation to something greater. And to this process, to this unfolding, I am fully committed.

As I walk this path of recovery, I am reminded that it is a path of transformation. Each step I take, each obstacle I overcome, each fear I face, brings me closer to the person I am meant to be. The person not defined by my addiction but by my courage, my resilience, and my capacity to change. I am reminded that in admitting my powerlessness, I have not lost anything. Instead, I have gained an understanding of myself and a connection with a power greater than myself that continues to guide me in my journey toward a fulfilling and sober life.

So, I persist in asking myself, am I willing to admit my powerlessness? Am I willing to allow a higher power to work within me? Am I willing to experience a mental change? And with each day, each moment, the answer becomes clearer and more resounding: Yes, I am willing. I am willing to continue this path, to embrace the journey, to live a life of recovery, one day at a time.

Taking these thoughts forward, I'd like to invite you to reflect on your own experiences. What areas in your life do you feel powerless over? Are there habits or thoughts that you find yourself returning to, despite their negative impact on your well-being? How might acknowledging this powerlessness be the first step toward change?

Moreover, how open are you to the idea of surrendering to a power greater than yourself? This doesn't necessarily have to be a religious or spiritual entity; it could be anything that you perceive as bigger and more powerful than your individual self. It could be nature, the universe, love, or the collective wisdom of those who have walked the path before you.

Are you ready to consider that this power might be a source of strength, guidance, and transformation? Are you willing to open your mind and heart to the possibility that this power could help bring about the internal shift necessary for recovery and growth?

Additionally, consider the concept of a mental change; a profound shift in perception and mindset. What does this mean to you? Are you willing to experience such a transformation? Do you believe it's possible for you? Remember, change isn't a one-time event but an ongoing process.

Are you willing to commit to this process, to this journey of self-discovery and transformation?

Reflect also on the idea of community and support. How open are you to seeking and accepting help from others? Do you see value in sharing your journey with those who can relate, who can offer insight, guidance, and empathetic understanding? How might engaging with a supportive community impact your path to recovery or growth?

Do you believe in your capacity to change? Despite the struggles, despite the setbacks, do you believe that you can overcome your challenges and build a life of fulfillment and well-being? Because belief in yourself, in your potential and your resilience, is perhaps the most crucial element in this journey.

Take a moment to sit with these questions. There are no right or wrong answers, only your truth. Your answers will provide valuable insight into your readiness for change and your approach to recovery or personal growth. Remember, every journey begins with a single step, and acknowledging where you are right now is the first step on this path. Are you ready to take it?

Once you have reflected on these questions, consider your responses and what they reveal about your current perspective on recovery, change, and personal growth. How does it resonate with your lived experience? How might these insights guide you in making decisions that align with your desire for growth and well-being?

The exploration doesn't stop here, though. As you walk this path, keep in mind that your journey is unique. It will unfold in its own time and in its own way. It's not about quick fixes or overnight transformations. It's about cultivating patience, perseverance, and compassion toward yourself.

Next, ask yourself what obstacles you foresee on this path? Is it fear? Is it a lack of confidence? Are there external factors that you perceive as hindrances? Identifying potential roadblocks ahead of time allows you to better prepare for them and develop strategies to overcome them.

Also, reflect on the resources you have available to you. These might include inner resources such as resilience, courage, and determination. They might also include external resources like supportive relationships, community groups, or professional guidance. How can you make the best use of these resources on your journey?

And while you're considering these resources, reflect on the role of gratitude in your life. How often do you take the time to appreciate the good things in your life? Gratitude has been shown to improve mental well-being, making it a valuable tool in your journey toward growth and recovery.

Consider, too, the role of self-care in your journey. Are you treating yourself with kindness? Are you giving yourself permission to rest, to feel, to falter? Recovery and growth aren't linear processes. They involve ups and downs, progress, and setbacks. During these times, self-care can provide the nurturing and resilience needed to keep moving forward.

These questions and reflections can provide valuable insights and guidance as you navigate your unique journey. They can help to frame your mindset, clarify your intentions, and empower your actions toward change and growth. Remember, this is your journey, and you have the power to shape it in ways that support your well-being and fulfillment. Are you ready to embark on this journey? Are you prepared to accept the challenges and embrace the possibilities that lie ahead?

Have you thought about the people you surround yourself with? Do they support your aspirations toward recovery and change, or do they hinder your progress, consciously or unconsciously? It's crucial to establish boundaries and surround yourself with individuals who respect and support your journey.

And how about forgiveness? Have you considered the power of forgiveness in your journey to recovery? This doesn't just mean forgiving others but also includes forgiving yourself for the mistakes and missteps you've made. Holding onto resentment and guilt only serves to hinder your progress. Can you work on cultivating forgiveness and letting go?

Next, think about how you handle stress. Stress is an inevitable part of life, and it's even more prevalent when you're working toward such a significant personal change. Have you developed effective stress management strategies? Could mindfulness, meditation, or physical exercise play a role in your stress management routine?

Additionally, consider your relationship with failure. Despite your best efforts, there will likely be setbacks on your journey. How do you view these moments of failure? Are they roadblocks, or can you view them as opportunities for learning and growth?

Moving forward, think about how much you trust the process. The path of recovery and change can be winding and unpredictable. Sometimes, it might feel like you're not moving at all. It's essential to have faith in the process and trust that even when progress isn't visible, it's happening beneath the surface.

Consider your vision for the future. Visualizing your journey's end can be a powerful motivator. What does recovery look like to you? What does growth feel like? Keeping this vision in mind can provide a sense of direction and hope, especially during challenging times.

Navigating the path of recovery is complex and deeply personal, but asking yourself these questions can provide insight and perspective. You are not alone on this journey, and it's okay to reach out for help when needed. Are you open to seeking and accepting help? How will you remind yourself of your strength and resilience when the path gets tough?

How do you perceive change? Change can be terrifying, but it is also the only constant in life. Fear of the unknown is a natural human reaction. Do you see change as a threat or can you reframe it as an opportunity to become a better version of yourself?

Next, ponder over the power of vulnerability. Do you consider vulnerability a strength or a weakness? Vulnerability is not a sign of weakness; it's a sign of strength. It takes courage to admit our shortcomings, to acknowledge our feelings, and to ask for help when we need it. Can you begin to appreciate your vulnerability as part of your authentic self?

Have you thought about your support system? As humans, we thrive on connection. Are you willing to reach out to others for support, whether it's family, friends, or a support group, and allow them to be there for you? Can you express your feelings and experiences honestly and openly with them?

Consider your relationship with yourself. Do you love and respect yourself? This is crucial because, ultimately, this journey is about you. Self-love and self-respect are essential in recovery. Are you kind to yourself when you stumble or do you beat yourself up over it?

Reflect on your personal boundaries. How well do you establish and maintain them? Maintaining personal boundaries is a way of communicating to others that you respect yourself. Can you say no when needed, even if it might disappoint others?

How is your relationship with patience? Change is often slow and gradual, almost imperceptible in the day-to-day. Are you willing to be patient with yourself and with the process?

Remember, there are no right or wrong answers to these questions. They are intended to prompt introspection and encourage self-awareness. This journey to recovery is uniquely yours, and every step, no matter how small, is a victory. Can you begin to view every day as an opportunity for growth, even if there are setbacks? Will you celebrate your small victories along the way, recognizing that they contribute to your larger journey? How will you remind yourself of the progress you've made when the road seems long and arduous

CHAPTER 2

UNDERSTANDING MY SITUATION

In the book of Alcoholics Anonymous, Dr. Silkworth breaks down the simplicity of understanding that addiction has two distinct parts. A disease of the body and an obsession of the mind. Let's discuss what Dr. Silkworth meant when he referred to alcoholism as an allergy.

When my mentor guided me through the book, he encouraged me to transform my personal experiences into questions. For instance, he asked, "Do you have an abnormal reaction to alcohol when you drink?" But before I could answer that question, I needed a clear understanding of what constitutes an "abnormal reaction." And my mentor shed light on it by illustrating the following scenarios.

"You know how alcoholics struggle to recall what happened the night before—where they were or who they were with? Have you noticed how they can never remember the conversations they had over the phone while drunk? They make bewildered calls at two a.m. and then again at ten a.m., seeking reassurance, asking, 'Are we okay?' This would be an example of an extreme. A reaction that normal drinkers do not have."

So, ask yourself: When you drink, do you have a normal or abnormal reaction? Is everything pleasant and ordinary, or do you find yourself regretting your actions while under the influence? Can you easily take or leave alcohol or drugs, stopping whenever you want? These introspective questions can help you discern the nature of your relationship with alcohol or drugs.

Dr. Silkworth also emphasized that the phenomenon of craving is exclusive to certain individuals and never occurs in average, moderate users. But what does craving truly mean? According to merriam-webster.com, it refers to a an intense, urgent, or abnormal desire or longing. When my mentor posed the question, "When you drink, do you crave more alcohol?" I found myself responding, "I don't know, but I always want more."

That, my friends, is precisely what craving entails. If every time you consume alcohol, you find yourself wanting for more, wouldn't you consider it a craving? It's essential to note that Alcoholics Anonymous primarily addresses alcoholism but its principles and insights can apply to any addiction, mental health crisis, or personal struggle. As we proceed, I encourage you to interpret the book in that broader context and apply its wisdom to your unique circumstances.

Dr. Silkworth stated that craving never manifests in the average, temperate drinker. When I read this sentence, it became abundantly clear to me that I was indeed an alcoholic. It wasn't just about the chaos, fear, and devastation I caused while drinking; it boiled down to the fact that whenever I consumed alcohol, everything about me changed drastically, departing from the realm of normalcy.

In the early days when the authors first shared their messages of hope, they delved into their inner experiences. They spoke about drinking alcohol and the insatiable desire for more. They touched upon the abnormal reactions to alcohol and the subsequent guilt, shame, and regret. They recounted their cycle of going to a hospital to detox, only to relapse again and again. They expressed feelings of hopelessness, fear, depression, and anxiety, the sense of life lacking purpose.

If you've attended Alcoholics Anonymous meetings, you might have encountered gatherings where individuals indulge in a great deal of seemingly pointless drama, recounting what are often referred to as "drunk-a-logs." Let me explain further.

As a newcomer, when you attend your first meeting, you seek a glimmer of hope. However, standing at the back of the room, you find yourself listening to a person rambling about their miserable, pathetic life. They talk about the wretched years spent in prison, the moment they achieved sobriety while locked in solitary confinement after assaulting another prisoner or guard. They share stories of numerous DUIs, drug-related encounters, encounters with law enforcement, repeated arrests, courtroom dramas, and time spent behind bars. These tales echo over and over again. They describe the challenges of probation, the exorbitant fees paid for legal representation and court fines. They mention their broken relationships, a spouse who has left them, and children who harbor resentment. They talk about bankruptcy, losing everything they had, and ending up homeless, defeated, and utterly alone. And then, amidst all the despair, they conclude with the words, "But hey, I'm grateful to be sober just for today."

As a newcomer, sitting in that room, feeling fearful and bewildered, if this is the only narrative you hear at your first meeting, you might start questioning, *Who are these people? I've never been to prison. I've never experienced solitary confinement. I would never harm another person in that way. I have no DUIs or arrests. I've never even had a conversation with a police officer or set foot in a courtroom. I still have a job. My spouse hasn't left me yet. My children might be worried, but I know they love me. I haven't reached the point of financial ruin. I'm not homeless, broken, defeated, and alone. However, I do acknowledge that I have a significant problem that I can't seem to control.*

In this situation, it's not surprising if the newcomer begins to doubt whether they truly have an addiction or alcoholism. They may think, *If this is what alcoholism looks like, maybe I'm not an alcoholic. I'm not like that person pouring their heart out up there.* And in that moment of doubt, they might get up and walk out, leaving behind the one place that should have been a safe haven. They leave behind the very space they needed most in that critical moment of their lives.

It's meant to be a place where we, as members, are meant to fulfill our duty and share a message of hope, not tales of misery and despair.

In this unfortunate scenario, we lose an individual before they even have a chance to understand what alcoholism truly means or discover their own identity within it. Through our ignorance and irresponsibility, we unintentionally snatch away their only fighting chance. Instead of fostering understanding and relatability, we create distance and confusion through stories of trauma that are better suited for discussions over a cup of coffee outside of AA rather than within the meeting rooms.

My mentor taught me the importance of always carrying a message of hope and encouragement when I attended a meeting. He reminded me that my purpose there was to identify those who needed to hear that there is indeed hope and to engage in conversations with them about it. He emphasized that if I felt compelled to share the pathetic and meaningless aspects of my life, I should do so in a coffee shop, not during an AA meeting.

So, let us remember the power of our words and the impact they can have on newcomers. Let us strive to create an atmosphere of hope, understanding, and support so that those who are seeking solace and guidance can find it within the rooms of Alcoholics Anonymous.

It is our responsibility to be mindful of the messages we convey in AA meetings. We should be aware of the newcomer's vulnerability and the courage it took for them to walk through those doors. It's crucial to offer them a sense of hope and a glimpse of what recovery can truly mean.

Instead of indulging in tales of misery and despair, we can share our experiences of transformation, personal growth, and the joy of living a sober life. We can speak about the newfound clarity, the mending of relationships, the rediscovery of passions, and the inner peace that comes with sobriety. By doing so, we offer newcomers a vision of what is possible for them.

Moreover, we must remember that the principles and teachings of the Twelve Steps extend beyond alcoholism. They can be applied to any addiction, mental health struggle, or personal challenge that individuals may face. Therefore, it is crucial to create an inclusive and understanding environment where everyone can find resonance and support, regardless of their specific circumstances.

When a newcomer enters those rooms, let us greet them with warmth and empathy. Let us share stories of hope, strength, and resilience. Let us emphasize that they are not alone in their journey and that recovery is possible. By embracing this approach, we foster an atmosphere that encourages newcomers to stay, to explore their own relationship with addiction or mental health, and to discover the path to a brighter future.

Ask yourself the question, "When I drink alcohol, do I crave more?" Dr. Silkworth stated that craving "never" occurs in the average drinker. But if you experience craving half the time you drink, it is likely that you are an alcoholic, according to Dr. Silkworth. He emphasizes that craving never happens in the average drinker.

The thing that distinguishes me from a non-alcoholic has nothing to do with the consequences of alcohol in my life, such as DUIs, arrests, divorce, and health issues. It all comes down to one thing: the phenomenon of craving. When I consume alcohol, I have an abnormal reaction—my face flushes, I break out in hives, and I want more. It's an allergic reaction.

Have you ever observed people who can have one or two drinks and then say, "I better slow down or stop"? I've witnessed this many times, but I can't relate to it. And what about those who don't finish their glass of wine or beer? In my world, that's absurd. That's just the beginning for me.

I've had friends question me about my drinking, asking why I can't just have a few drinks and leave it at that. Even my close friend, who was dying from cancer, couldn't understand why I couldn't have just one last drink with him. He could drink without losing control, while I always ended up a mess.

Dr. Silkworth describes how alcoholics become irritable, restless, and discontent unless they can have more alcohol. They see others drink without a problem, but for them, the craving takes over, leading to a cycle of drinking until they pass out. This also applies to sobriety. I need to find things in sobriety that replace the role of drinking, or else I'll become irritable, restless, and discontent, which will eventually lead me back to drinking. The Twelve Steps offer peace, calm, and hope.

In the past, I hid alcohol all around my house, afraid of running out or being caught by my wife and kids. I would tell them I was only drinking wine but secretly sneak vodka from a hidden bottle. It didn't matter that I passed out early or faced consequences; once I had that first drink, everything seemed fine.

Interestingly, the same experience exists in sobriety. If I follow the Steps, I have the assurance that, as long as I stay sober, I'll be happy and everything will be okay.

Dr. Silkworth emphasizes the need for an entire mental change to have any hope of recovery. This change starts with altering the way we think.

If I had the power to change my thinking about alcohol and drinking without any help, I wouldn't need the Twelve Steps, a higher power, or a mentor. But the reality is, I can't do it on my own.

To experience an essential psychic change, I need something beyond human power. Mentors, spouses, material possessions, or external factors can't bring about this change.

In "Bill's Story" from The Big Book, Bill Wilson realizes he has no power to stop drinking on his own when his friend Ebby visits him sober. This is the essence of Step One: recognizing that human power alone is insufficient to overcome the problem.

Step One isn't just about not drinking or using drugs; it's about acknowledging that I have no power to stop on my own. More information or techniques won't solve the problem. Until I found the Twelve Steps and experienced a spiritual awakening, I was bound to continue drinking and using drugs.

If I could drink without any consequences, would I still be drinking? Am I seeking sobriety because I genuinely want to stop drinking, or am I trying to escape the suffering and pain that come with it?

For a long time, I attended AA meetings while still drinking. I kept going, even though I was often drunk and didn't talk to anyone. Looking back, I realize it was because I wanted to end the pain and suffering in my life. I had reached my breaking point. But I hadn't fully accepted the fact that I had no power over alcohol.

Understanding Step One goes beyond simply admitting that I'm a drunk. It's about recognizing that I have no power to stop drinking and stay sober. I may want to be sober, but I can't stop on my own.

In Bill's story, he becomes open to change when he realizes that neither he nor his friend Ebby have any power. They both lack the ability to control their drinking once they start and face the phenomenon of craving.

I hadn't fully grasped the true meaning of Step One. I thought it was about admitting I was an alcoholic, but it was much deeper than that. It meant acknowledging that my life had become unmanageable and that my main problem lay in my thinking. Alcohol was just a symptom of a much larger issue.

Consider your own life experiences. Was your thinking clear or clouded before embarking on the Twelve Steps? It's important to recognize that addiction is a real disease, just like cancer or diabetes. If we were diagnosed with a physical ailment, we would seek help and gather information. Similarly, we must understand who we truly are and what we're dealing with before we can move forward and seek assistance.

Reflect on your own behavior:
Have you ever drunk or used drugs alone when you felt ashamed and didn't want to?
Have you consumed alcohol alone when you were feeling good or didn't feel anything at all?
Have you used alcohol to numb your emotions or to seek a feeling?
Have you ever drunk or used drugs because you just had to feel something?

The authors of The Big Book explain that moderate drinkers can easily give up alcohol if they have a strong reason to do so. They can take it or leave it.

Ask yourself:

Can I take or leave alcohol? If you can, then you're likely a moderate drinker rather than an alcoholic. However, there are individuals known as hard drinkers who struggle to moderate or stop drinking, even with sufficient reasons. They may require medical attention to address their problematic habits.

Evaluate whether you have sufficient reasons to stop or moderate your drinking at this point in your life. Are you truly a hard drinker?

In my own journey, I believed I was just a hard drinker. I would rationalize my excessive drinking by thinking I deserved it after working hard. I even prioritized alcohol over my marriage and family, unwilling to give it up. But in retrospect, the chaos and unmanageability of my life should have made it clear that I wasn't just a hard drinker.

What sets a real alcoholic apart is the loss of control over the amount they consume once they start drinking. One drink is never enough. I resonate with this distinction because I lose all control over alcohol once I take that first sip. I can't stop, no matter the consequences.

Sobriety, for me, means abstaining from all drugs, including alcohol and tobacco. Nicotine is still a drug, and I acknowledge that sobriety entails total abstinence. Others may have their own experiences and define sobriety differently, attending meetings that align with their needs.

The Big Book discusses the mental obsession that plagues alcoholics. Our main problem lies in our thinking, making alcohol just a symptom. It's critical to examine the state of our thinking before starting the Twelve Steps.

Ask yourself, "Was my thinking clear or clouded prior to beginning the Twelve Steps?"

If we are honest with ourselves, we will likely realize that our thinking was clouded, distorted, and consumed by the obsession to drink or use drugs. Our minds were constantly preoccupied with obtaining and consuming our substance of choice. We may have made promises to ourselves to cut back or quit, but those promises were quickly broken as soon as the craving took hold.

Step One is not solely about admitting that we are alcoholics or addicts, it goes much deeper than that. It's about acknowledging the powerlessness and unmanageability in our lives. It's recognizing that our thinking is fundamentally flawed when it comes to substances.

I remember hearing someone at a meeting confidently proclaim, "I'm a real alcoholic." At the time, I couldn't understand why they would emphasize that point. Weren't we all alcoholics or addicts in the room? Little did I know that an alcoholic could start off as a moderate drinker or drug user. The difference lies in the loss of control once we take that first drink or drug. We are unable to stop or moderate; one is never enough.

Reflect on your own experiences:
Can you stop drinking or using drugs once you start, despite the consequences?
Are you able to control the mental obsession once you've taken that first drink or drug?

For me, Step One was not just a matter of confessing that I was an alcoholic, it was a profound realization that my life had become completely unmanageable. I couldn't rely on my own willpower or human power to conquer my addiction. My thinking was flawed, and no amount of information or techniques would bring about lasting sobriety.

To truly recover, we need to undergo a mental shift—a profound transformation in the way we think and perceive the world. This change cannot be achieved through human effort alone; it requires something greater than ourselves.

Ask yourself, "Can a mentor, spouse, or material possessions bring about this essential internal change in me?"

For me, the answer is a resounding no. No external influence or material possession can provide the necessary transformation required for me to change. We must be open to the possibility that we need something beyond human power—a spiritual solution—to experience this personal revolution.

In Bill's story found in the book of Alcoholics Anonymous, he comes to this realization when he recognizes that neither he nor his friend possesses any power to control their drinking. They are both powerless and devoid of any effective solution. This realization is at the heart of Step One—acknowledging that no human power can restore us to sanity or alleviate our addiction.

Step One is not about mere abstinence from drinking or using drugs for a day. It's about surrendering our illusion of control and recognizing the need for a power greater than ourselves. It's about embracing the fact that we are entirely powerless and that our lives have become unmanageable.

So, as you continue your journey through the Twelve Steps, keep in mind that Step One is not just about stopping drinking or using. It's about acknowledging the depths of powerlessness and unmanageability in our lives. It's about seeking a spiritual solution and embarking on a transformative path toward recovery.

Remember, you are not alone in this journey. Many have traveled the same path and found freedom from addiction through the Twelve Steps. With openness, willingness, and a commitment to change, you can find a new way of life—one that is free from the grips of addiction and filled with hope, serenity, and lasting sobriety.

As you go deeper into your understanding of Step One, it's important to address another crucial aspect: the ability to take or leave alcohol. This concept can shed further light on the nature of your relationship with substances.

This distinction is what separates a real alcoholic or addict from a moderate or hard drinker. The inability to stop or control one's consumption once it begins is a defining characteristic of addiction. It's a clear indicator that our relationship with substances has transcended the boundaries of normalcy. Ask yourself: "Can I genuinely take or leave alcohol or drugs?"

If you can comfortably and effortlessly moderate your use, it suggests that you may fall into the category of a moderate or hard drinker. However, if you find yourself unable to stop or moderate, despite the negative consequences or you find that there is no sufficient reason left that can stop you, it's likely that you are facing the challenges of the disease of addiction.

In my own experience, I used to convince myself that I was just a hard drinker. I believed that my hard work entitled me to indulge in excessive drinking. When confronted by my wife about my drinking problem, I prioritized alcohol over my relationship. Looking back, it becomes evident that my life had become unmanageable and that my drinking was far from normal.

Recognizing the distinction between a hard drinker and a real alcoholic or addict is vital. Understanding that taking one sip of alcohol or one dose of a drug triggers an uncontrollable craving and loss of control is crucial in acknowledging the severity of our condition.

Step One requires us to be clear about our own experiences and honest with ourselves. It is not about conforming to a label but about understanding the depth of our powerlessness and unmanageability. It's about acknowledging that our addiction is not solely about the substances themselves but about the distorted thinking and obsession that consumes us.

By embracing Step One and surrendering to the reality of our powerlessness, we open the door to a new way of living. We can embark on a path of recovery, guided by the Twelve Steps and the support of others who have faced similar challenges.

Remember, you are not defined by your past actions or mistakes. Step One invites you to confront your addiction head-on and seek the help and guidance needed to experience a profound psychic change. Through honesty, willingness, and an open mind, you can find freedom from the grip of addiction and discover a life filled with serenity, purpose, and lasting sobriety.

Consider this analogy: If you were diagnosed with lung cancer, would you continue smoking without seeking assistance or learning about how to quit? Probably not. Similarly, we need to recognize the seriousness of our addiction and the necessity of seeking help and support.

Now, let's explore a significant realization that had a profound impact on me when I first encountered it:

Addiction is not limited to a specific substance; it encompasses the entire spectrum of mind-altering substances. Whether it's alcohol, tobacco, cocaine, opiates, heroin, methamphetamine, or benzodiazepines, the underlying principle remains the same. It's crucial to examine our own experiences honestly.

For instance, I admitted that alcohol was my drug of choice, but I also acknowledged that I had a propensity for using any substance that could produce a high. Once I started, there was never enough, and the phenomenon of craving took control.

We must emphasize that the alcoholic's main problem lies in their mind rather than their body. Alcohol or drugs are merely symptoms of a deeper issue—our distorted thinking and obsession. This understanding prompts us to reflect on our thought patterns and the manageability of our lives. Ask yourself: Before starting the Twelve Steps, was your thinking clear or obscured?

When I honestly evaluated my own situation, I realized that my thinking was clouded by my addiction. My ability to reason, make sound decisions, and lead a manageable life was compromised. Chaos and confusion seemed to follow me wherever I went.

Step One compels us to confront the reality of our powerlessness. It challenges the notion that we can control our drinking or drug use once we start. It exposes the illusion of managing our addiction without external assistance. It's about recognizing that our best efforts to control or stop using on our own have been futile.

Bill's story in the book of Alcoholics Anonymous exemplifies this awakening. He reaches a point of openness when he acknowledges that neither he nor his friend Ebby possessed any power over their addiction. This realization becomes the essence of Step One: recognizing that no human power alone can relieve us of our addiction or solve the complexities of our lives.

It's important to remember that Step One isn't solely about admitting we are powerless over alcohol or drugs. It's about recognizing the unmanageability that has permeated our lives as a result of our addiction. By acknowledging our powerlessness, we become willing to seek a power greater than ourselves to guide us toward recovery.

As you explore Step One further, continue to reflect on your own experiences and evaluate the manageability of your life. Seek honesty within yourself and be open to the possibility of a psychic change. Through humility, surrender, and a willingness to embrace a new way of living, you can embark on the transformative journey of recovery and find a life free from the grip of addiction.

Step One requires us to examine the manageability of our lives in the face of addiction. It urges us to honestly evaluate the chaos, turmoil, and consequences that have accompanied our substance abuse. It is an opportunity to confront the stark reality of our powerlessness and unmanageability.

Ask yourself:

How manageable has my life been while in the grip of addiction? Have I experienced repeated negative consequences, damaged relationships, financial instability, legal issues, or emotional turmoil?

For me, the answer was clear. My addiction had made my life completely unmanageable. Despite my best intentions and fleeting moments of control, I always found myself back in the vicious cycle of craving, indulgence, and suffering.

Step One illuminates the fundamental truth that we cannot overcome addiction through sheer willpower or human effort alone. No matter how determined we may be, we are powerless over our addiction. This admission may initially feel disheartening, but it opens the door to a new path of recovery.

The essence of Step One lies in fully conceding to our innermost self that we have the disease of addiction or mental illness, surrendering to the fact that our lives have become unmanageable and that we cannot conquer addiction on our own. It is an invitation to let go of our self-reliance and embrace the support, guidance, and strength that come from a power greater than ourselves.

Ask yourself, "Am I willing to concede first to my addiction? Am I willing to let go of the illusion of control and surrender to a higher power, which can restore me to sanity and provide the necessary foundation for my recovery?"

Accepting our powerlessness does not mean we are weak or hopeless. On the contrary, it signifies strength, humility, and a willingness to embark on a transformative journey. By embracing Step One, we create space for the necessary mental change to occur within us.

This change is not a mere intellectual understanding but a profound shift in our thinking, attitude, and perspective. It is a transformation that allows us to let go of our old patterns of behavior, distorted thinking, and destructive habits. It opens the door to a new way of living and experiencing life—one that is guided by spiritual principles, self-awareness, and a commitment to growth.

In the journey of recovery, Step One lays the foundation for the subsequent steps and the transformative process that follows. It invites us to explore our own experiences, confront our powerlessness, and be willing to seek a power beyond ourselves.

Remember, Step One is not a one-time realization but an ongoing practice of humility, surrender, and self-reflection. As we continue to work the steps, we deepen our understanding of our powerlessness and unmanageability while embracing the strength and support of a higher power and the fellowship of others in recovery.

With each step forward, we move closer to a life of serenity, freedom, and authentic connection. The journey begins with Step One—the crucial gateway to a new way of living.

CHAPTER 3

EXPLORING THE TRUTH IN STEP ONE

If I am willing to accept the truth found in step one, it might just set me free. The first step is a profound and powerful acknowledgment of one's own powerlessness over alcohol. This can be a challenging concept to grasp, especially considering our societal emphasis on control and autonomy. However, this admission is a crucial cornerstone in the journey toward recovery.

In the context of addiction, acknowledging powerlessness is not about accepting defeat or giving up. Rather, it's an honest recognition of the reality of one's situation. It's a realization that our attempts to control our alcohol use have been unsuccessful and that our lives, as a result, have become unmanageable. It's about admitting that we are caught in a destructive cycle that we can't break on our own.

This admission serves as a catalyst for change. It helps us break free from denial and confront the reality of our addiction head-on. In many ways, this step is about surrendering—not to the addiction but to the truth of our situation. It's about letting go of our illusions of control and acknowledging that our willpower alone is not enough to overcome the addiction.

Embracing powerlessness is a step toward empowerment. By acknowledging our powerlessness, we create a space for growth and transformation. We start to understand that our power doesn't lie in our ability to control everything but in our ability to adapt, learn, and grow from our experiences.

I was aware that my thinking had become obscured, clouding my mind and causing me immense pain, suffering, financial struggles, and legal troubles. The authors I read shared an understanding that many alcoholics, without comprehending why, lose their ability to choose once they take that first drink. I can certainly relate to this, can you?

Throughout this chapter, we will delve into the application of Step One, which requires us to admit our powerlessness over alcohol. Let's pause and transform this into a question: Do we lose the power to choose when we consume alcohol or drugs?

In meetings, I often hear people say, "I choose not to drink today." But if it were truly a matter of choice, wouldn't I be able to abstain without the need for AA, the Twelve Steps, mentors, or a higher power? If it were that simple, I would just refrain from drinking!

Years ago, my brother started drinking wine, but he managed to stop when he realized it was interfering with his work and family. Does he sound like a real alcoholic? I don't think so. If I had that kind of control, I would do the same. So why was it so challenging for me to quit? I learned that, as someone with alcoholism, willpower is practically nonexistent. We struggle to remember the extent of our past suffering and humiliation, which would deter us from taking that first drink.

In other words, merely recalling the severity of my experiences isn't sufficient enough reason to prevent me from drinking again. Regardless of how much knowledge, suffering, or pain I accumulate, I cannot maintain sobriety. Even the potential loss of my loved ones, friends, business, marriage, children, and the certainty of health issues cannot dissuade me. Nothing seems capable of preventing me from drinking.

It is vital for my well-being that I admit, deep within myself, that once I start drinking, I have no control. That I have the disease of addiction. I must surrender to the fact that there is absolutely nothing I can do to stay sober and I will inevitably keep drinking no matter what. I have no defense against the consequences that follow that first drink.

Let's ask ourselves, "Do we have any defense against the first drink?" What does that even mean? It doesn't mean that I have no defense prior to taking the drink. It means that once I take the first drink, I have no defense against the next.

Once again, the authors stress that alcoholics are powerless once they take that first sip. And for me, this has always been true. I needed power more than anything to refrain from drinking. I needed something greater than myself—a higher power that possesses real strength and real power. And I needed it right now! Not six months later. Right now!

In the past, I believed that attending AA meetings or seeking treatment would equip me with the tools to stop drinking. That's what I had been led to believe. However, I didn't realize at the time that what I truly needed was to experience my First Step. I had never genuinely taken it before. I had to surrender and acknowledge that I had no power. I needed to admit, as the Twelve Steps outline, that I am "powerless" once I consume alcohol, defenseless against the overwhelming craving that follows.

There is no question that AA and NA meetings work for recovery. This has been true from the beginning of meetings in 1934 in Akron Ohio. Then why does AA and NA fail for so many? Why did it have an 85-90% success rate for everyone attending meetings starting in 1934 and now has just the opposite. Why does AA and NA only work for about 5-10%?

Let's examine the possibility that a significant number of individuals attending meetings of Alcoholics Anonymous (AA), Narcotics Anonymous (NA), Cocaine Anonymous (CA), and other support groups may never truly experience Step One or continue on to work all twelve steps to completion. It raises the question of whether it becomes easier for them to rely on meeting attendance to stay sober rather than undertaking the work required in Step One.

Could it be that attending meetings becomes a convenient substitute for the rigorous self-reflection, admission of powerlessness over the disease and work demanded by Step One? By attending meetings regularly and seeking solace in the fellowship, individuals may find a sense of stability and support without having to confront the depths of their addiction and the unmanageability it has caused in their lives.

If this is the case, it raises concerns about the long-term efficacy of such an approach. Does relying solely on daily meetings, asking a higher power to keep me sober one day at a time, truly address the underlying issues of addiction and unmanageability? Is it enough to manage the disease daily without delving into the root causes and making a genuine commitment to personal transformation?

When we examine the wording of the Twelve Steps, we see that Step One explicitly requires a specific admission and surrender process. It demands fully conceding to our innermost selves that we have a disease of addiction and acknowledging the unmanageability it has brought upon us. Without this deep self-awareness and surrender, it becomes challenging to move forward in the steps.

Step Two follows with coming to believe in the existence of a higher power that can restore us to sanity. Step Three then calls for a decision to turn our lives over to this higher power, relinquishing our attempts at managing the disease on our own. These steps build upon the foundation of Step One, where we must first recognize our powerlessness and unmanageability.

If one attends meetings every day, seeking divine assistance just to stay sober one day at a time, but fails to fully concede that they have a disease of addiction and that their life has become unmanageable, the question arises: What are the chances of staying sober and free? Is it not merely buying time and engaging in a daily recovery routine without addressing the underlying issues?

It is important to acknowledge that while attending meetings and relying on a higher power can be valuable components of a recovery journey, they alone may not lead to lasting sobriety. To increase the likelihood of staying sober, it is crucial to engage in the transformative work of the Twelve Steps, including a profound Step One experience.

By working through the steps and fully surrendering to a higher power, individuals open themselves up to a process of healing, growth, and self-discovery. They gain the tools and insights necessary to address the root causes of addiction, develop healthier coping mechanisms, and cultivate a spiritual connection that supports their recovery.

While regular meeting attendance and reliance on a higher power are beneficial aspects of recovery, it is essential to go beyond these surface-level approaches. Engaging in the deep self-analysis, admission of powerlessness, and surrender required in Step One lays the foundation for a profound and transformative recovery journey. By fully embracing the Twelve Steps, individuals increase their chances of achieving lasting sobriety and freedom from the grip of addiction.

By neglecting the crucial work of Step One and solely depending on meeting attendance, individuals may find themselves merely treading water in their recovery. While attending meetings can provide temporary relief and support, it may not address the fundamental issues that contribute to addiction and hinder long-term sobriety.

Without fully embracing Step One, individuals may miss out on the opportunity to confront the destructive nature of their addiction and acknowledge the need for a higher power to guide their recovery. By failing to concede that they have a disease of addiction and that their life has become unmanageable, they risk remaining trapped in a cycle of temporary relief without addressing the underlying causes of their addictive behaviors.

When individuals attend meetings every day, year after year, relying on the hope that a higher power will keep them sober just for today, they may unwittingly be avoiding the necessary work of self-reflection, personal growth, and transformative change. By not fully committing to the steps, they may find themselves in a state of complacency, merely going through the motions of recovery without experiencing true freedom from their addiction.

While it is commendable to develop a recovery plan and engage in a daily routine, it is important to recognize that these actions alone may not be sufficient for sustainable sobriety. Without actively working through the Twelve Steps, individuals may miss out on the profound healing and self-discovery that can occur when they confront their addiction head-on and embrace a new way of life.

Working through the steps offers individuals an opportunity to identify and address the underlying issues, trauma, and patterns of behavior that contribute to their addictive tendencies. It provides a framework for personal growth, spiritual connection, and the development of healthier coping mechanisms. Each step builds upon the previous one, guiding individuals toward a more meaningful and fulfilling life in recovery.

While the journey through the Twelve Steps may be challenging and require self-examination and vulnerability, it is through this process that individuals can experience profound transformation and lasting freedom from addiction. By fully committing to Step One and progressing through the subsequent steps, individuals increase their chances of not only staying sober but also experiencing a newfound sense of purpose, fulfillment, and inner peace.

By undergoing a First Step experience, admitting my powerlessness, and conceding to my innermost self, I was finally able to surrender and discover a power greater than myself. Once I surrendered, I developed an intense desire to seek genuine power—a power that is authentic.

Before this personal experience, I was not inclined to seek a power greater than myself. Consider this: If I already possessed the power necessary to stop drinking and maintain sobriety, would I require a First Step experience? I should be capable of quitting whenever I desire. That's precisely why the authors dedicate forty-three pages of their book to Step One—it is the most crucial step.

The Twelve Steps help us discern whether we are unable to drink in moderation or if complete abstinence is necessary. The question we need to ask ourselves is, "Can I control my drinking once I start?"

For some individuals, moderation is possible. They can have a few drinks and stop without it spiraling into a destructive pattern. However, for others, like myself, once we start drinking, all bets are off. Our ability to control and moderate our intake goes out the window. We find ourselves caught in a cycle of craving and compulsion, unable to stop until we are completely intoxicated.

This lack of control over our drinking is a significant indicator of our powerlessness. It shows that we are unable to manage alcohol in a way that is safe and healthy. Despite our best intentions, we consistently find ourselves succumbing to the allure of alcohol and losing control over our consumption.

Through the process of self-reflection and honest introspection, we can gain a deeper understanding of our relationship with alcohol. We can examine our past experiences and behaviors to recognize the patterns of powerlessness and loss of control. This self-understanding is crucial in accepting our powerlessness and surrendering to the truth.

In the recovery journey, Step One guides us to confront this reality head-on. It encourages us to let go of our ego and pride and admit that we cannot conquer our alcoholism through sheer willpower. We must acknowledge that our attempts to control our drinking have been futile and that we need a power greater than ourselves to restore us to sanity.

It is essential to remember that admitting powerlessness is not a sign of weakness. On the contrary, it takes immense strength and courage to face the truth about ourselves and confront our limitations. By embracing our powerlessness, we open ourselves up to the possibility of finding a higher power and a solution that goes beyond our own understanding.

Through the process of surrender, acceptance, and seeking a power greater than ourselves, we can embark on a transformative journey of recovery. This journey involves working through the Twelve Steps, seeking support from others who have walked a similar path, and developing a spiritual connection that helps us maintain sobriety and find meaning in our lives.

Ultimately, Step One serves as the foundation for our recovery. It is the starting point that sets us on a path of self-discovery, healing, and growth. By acknowledging our powerlessness and embracing the truth, we open ourselves up to the possibility of a new way of living—one that is free from the grip of alcohol and filled with hope, serenity, and purpose.

With Step One, we have delved into the depths of powerlessness and unmanageability. We have acknowledged the patterns of our addictive behaviors, the loss of control, and the havoc they have wreaked upon our lives. Now, as we move forward, we must confront the question of what lies beyond our powerlessness.

Many of us may have initially believed that simply attending meetings or seeking external solutions would be enough to overcome our addiction. We may have thought that gaining knowledge or relying on willpower alone would be sufficient to break free from the grip of alcohol or drugs. However, as we have come to realize, these superficial approaches often fall short.

Step One challenges us to question whether a middle-of-the-road solution, such as attending meetings without actively engaging in the work required, can truly lead to lasting sobriety. We are urged to reflect upon the individuals we may have encountered in recovery settings who continually attend meetings but fail to experience true transformation. These individuals may carry resentment, resist personal growth, and rely on external rituals without delving into the deeper work of the Twelve Steps.

If we find ourselves in a similar position, going through the motions without a genuine commitment to self-reflection and spiritual development, we must recognize that this approach is unlikely to yield lasting results. We need to confront the truth that genuine recovery requires more than mere attendance; it necessitates active engagement, personal introspection, and a sincere willingness to do the necessary work.

For me, I walked that path of half-hearted engagement for several years. I attended countless meetings, listened to the stories, and sought solace in the camaraderie of others. However, I neglected to take the vital step of surrendering to a higher power and fully immersing myself in the Twelve Steps. I clung to the illusion that I had the power within myself to conquer addiction, failing to recognize that my willpower alone was insufficient.

It was only when I experienced my personal rock-bottom, a place of complete powerlessness and desperation of a dying man, that I fully conceding to my addiction and truly surrendered. In that moment of surrender, I realized that my own self-will had led me astray, and I needed to seek a power greater than myself to guide me toward a new way of life.

Step One paves the way for Step Two, where we embark on a journey of faith and spirituality. It invites us to explore the possibility of a higher power that can restore us to sanity. This higher power can manifest in various forms—whether it be a traditional religious deity, a universal energy, or a collective wisdom found within the recovery community. The key is to find a power greater than ourselves that we can trust and rely upon.

As we move forward, we must be willing to shed our skepticism and open ourselves up to the potential of a spiritual awakening. This requires humility, openness, and a willingness to let go of our preconceived notions. By embracing Step One's admission of powerlessness and unmanageability, we create the necessary space within ourselves to welcome a higher power and its transformative influence.

CHAPTER 4

CONFRONTING THE DEBTS OF UNMANAGEABILITY

The concept of rock bottom is frequently discussed in the context of addiction and mental illness. It's a phrase that we encounter often, and we may even use it to describe our own experiences, believing that we have hit rock bottom only to realize that it was merely another rung on the downward spiral. We deceive ourselves into thinking that it's the ultimate low, but in reality it's just a new level of acceptability, a point where we can momentarily escape the anguish by self-medicating.

Rock bottom is more than just a catchy phrase; it's a symbolic representation of the depths to which one can sink when trapped in the throes of addiction or mental illness. It signifies a state of utter despair, hopelessness, and desolation. It's the point where the consequences of our actions, the wreckage of our lives, and the weight of our struggles become undeniable.

But here's the harsh truth: rock bottom isn't a singular event or a fixed destination. It's a fluid and subjective experience that varies from person to person. What may be rock bottom for one individual might not be for another. Each of us has our own unique journey, and our personal rock bottom is an individualized, deeply personal threshold.

The danger lies in the illusion of acceptability. When we find ourselves in a new low, a place where we can momentarily numb the pain through self-medication, we convince ourselves that it's manageable, tolerable even. We mask our emotions, drown out the turmoil, and pretend that everything is under control. We become adept at justifying our destructive behavior, finding solace in the temporary relief it provides.

Yet, this deceptive cycle of self-medication only perpetuates our descent. By numbing our pain, we deny ourselves the opportunity to confront the root causes of our addiction or mental illness. We delay the necessary healing and transformation that can only occur when we confront the truth head-on.

True rock bottom isn't about reaching an acceptable low. It's about reaching a breaking point, an internal shift that shatters our illusions of control and pushes us to seek a way out. It's the moment when we confront the devastating consequences of our actions, acknowledge the depths of our pain, and realize that we can no longer sustain this destructive path.

Rock bottom is not a place to linger but a pivotal moment for change. It's the catalyst that propels us toward recovery, healing, and a newfound determination to reclaim our lives. It's the starting point of a long and arduous journey, where we must confront our demons, face our vulnerabilities, and embrace the difficult but transformative work of recovery.

The profound significance of Step One lies in the acknowledgment that one's life has become unmanageable. To truly grasp the gravity of this admission, it is essential to delve into the realm of our most irrational and bewildering actions. Beyond the obvious consequences like DUIs, arrests, and public embarrassments, we must explore the deeper layers of insanity that addiction can manifest.

Allow me to share my personal experience. It occurred when I had already achieved four years of sobriety, actively participating in meetings, mentoring others, and diligently working the Twelve Steps. At that point, I believed I had attained the pinnacle of happiness and success in my recovery. I had become synonymous with AA, adorned with rings, hats, and t-shirts proudly proclaiming "RECOVERY." I chaired a meeting every day and served as a secretary for another in the evenings. I convinced myself that I had everything under control.

One fateful day, while dining with a friend at a convention in Las Vegas, he offered me a glass of wine. In that pivotal moment, my mind whispered, *Perhaps I can handle a glass of wine today. I've got this.* Can you sense the insanity in this line of thinking? Does it depict a life that is manageable or unmanageable? Is it the behavior of a person living in normalcy or abnormality? Despite years of relentless pursuit to find sobriety, enduring multiple treatment programs and achieving four years of uninterrupted abstinence, my mind was audaciously suggesting, *Go ahead, Cord; you can handle it.* How deluded I was!

The point to be grasped here is that, even after four years of struggling toward a full freedom, I was nowhere close to experiencing true recovery. Genuine, long-lasting sobriety demands effort and commitment. It necessitates a complete journey through the Twelve Steps, a process I had neglected at that point. Instead, I found myself living each day by sheer willpower, white knuckling through, attending meetings, acquiring a mentor, reading Alcoholics Anonymous, and perpetually engaged in my Fourth Step. However, I had not yet mentored anyone because I had not truly embraced the transformative power of the Steps. I relied on prayers, asking God to keep me sober "just for today." I was living under the assumption that this was my identity because that's what I had been instructed to do. It was a pitiful existence destined for failure.

Since I had not worked through all the Twelve Steps, I lacked genuine sobriety. A single drink had the power to plunge me back into the abyss, eradicating all the progress I had made over those four years. One tiny drink, and I lost the power to choose. I had no defense. It was worse than ever before. One small sip of alcohol sent me spiraling out of control, causing me to lose everything I had gained. Days later, I awoke in a golf resort in Scottsdale, Arizona, bewildered and unaware of how I had even arrived there, surrounded by nine, empty ½-gallon vodka bottles scattered throughout the room. I continued my self-destructive drinking spree for the next two years!

Can you fathom the depths of unmanageability displayed here?

The Big Book of Alcoholics Anonymous aptly describes the concept of "unmanageability" in Step Two. It encompasses difficulties in relationships, a lack of emotional control, financial troubles, an inability to sustain a livelihood, constant fear, a profound sense of uselessness, genuine unhappiness, and a disconnection from God or a higher power.

To assess your own manageability, answer the following questions with a simple YES or NO:

Am I currently struggling in my relationships?
Can I maintain control over my temper and emotions?
Do I feel worthless and devoid of purpose?
Am I plagued by depression, anxiety, and misery?
Do I hold the job that truly fulfills me?
Is fear a constant presence in my life?
Am I genuinely unhappy?
Do I rely on daily prayers, seeking God's assistance to stay sober only for today?
Am I capable of making a positive impact on others?

The mental obsession associated with alcoholism extends beyond the desire for a drink. It manifests in various rationalizations detailed within The Big Book, which enable the alcoholic to continue their destructive behavior. These may include switching from hard liquor to beer or wine, imposing restrictions like not drinking until after five p.m., or attempting to limit the amount of alcohol one purchases and keeps. The book even recounts a story of an individual adding whiskey to milk, believing that consuming it with other liquids would lessen its impact. Such behavior is undeniably absurd, wouldn't you agree?

Returning to my ill-advised act in Las Vegas, we must question whether my reaction to that drink was normal or abnormal. Undeniably, it was abnormal. I experienced the phenomenon of craving. Once I took that initial sip, no rational justification could compel me to remain sober. It was game over! I lost all control the moment I started drinking. I forfeited the power to choose.

It is crucial to acknowledge that the fundamental requirement for progress lies in conceding our powerlessness. As long as we cling to any notion that suggests we have control, no other approach will work. This is an indisputable truth of the disease. If you believe that more knowledge, more meetings, a better mentor, an improved book, innovative technology, or medication alone will suffice to keep you sober, you are mistaken.

Merely telling yourself, *I need more information, that's it, just more information, and I'll stay sober,* is futile. Without grasping this concept, you cannot proceed to Step Two, which leads us to a power greater than ourselves, capable of transforming our thinking. Therefore, if you still cling to the idea that anything else can preserve your sobriety, there is no room to progress. This is precisely what happened to me for several years.

During that time, I wandered between seven different treatment centers, programs, and AA meetings, constantly seeking more information. I refused to concede to my innermost self that I had an addiction and my life had become unmanageable, that I had lost all control, that I was powerless, and that I could not stop drinking once I started. I denied the truth. My actions during that period serve as undeniable proof of my resistance. Without power, I would inevitably drink every day, regardless of any other circumstance.

Hence, the only approach that truly works is to fully concede in acknowledging, "I am powerless to stop." Additionally, it necessitates a commitment to daily prayer and meditation, conducting regular self-assessments, and actively working through the Twelve Steps. For me, engaging in addiction services at my treatment center and aiding others became the sole path to maintaining sobriety.

To conclude Step One, answer the following critical questions with a resolute YES or NO:

Am I willing to concede to my innermost self that I am an alcoholic or addict?

Am I willing to concede that I lack the power to quit once I start?

Do I acknowledge that my life has become unmanageable due to my addiction?

I hope you will experience your own profound Step One awakening. At this moment, you might not feel particularly good about yourself. Perhaps you sense your life spiraling out of control, engulfed in unmanageability and powerlessness, convinced that you will continue drinking no matter what. Feelings of queasiness, despair, fear, and anxiety may consume you.

Allow me to share a glimpse of my own initial Step One experience. Please understand that I share this not to recount my past transgressions but to offer you insight into what you might encounter and what to aspire to. As you embark on this journey, you may not feel the bottom yet, but don't lose hope.

REACHING THE DEPTHS OF THE ABYSS:

During the peak of my drinking, my life had descended into such chaos and unmanageability that one might believe it was a fabrication or an impossibility. It was an absolute train wreck.

I had always been the epitome of control, boasting wealth, a luxurious home, new cars, and the respect of those who worked with and for me. I can't recall the exact moment when everything started spiraling out of control, but when it did, it resembled a flaming 747 hurtling from the sky, unstoppable and catastrophic.

My battle with alcoholism spanned over two decades, but within a year, everything crumbled before me. Due to my drinking and the ensuing financial turmoil, my wife left, taking our daughter with her. My business associates disavowed me, and my once-thriving enterprise collapsed, leaving me bankrupt. Legal issues, DUIs, courtrooms, and jail time ensued.

I vividly remember the day my wife walked out, leaving me utterly alone. I sat on the couch, fixated on the television, drowning my sorrows in alcohol. I had never experienced such anguish, despair, and loneliness before. The more I drank, the more I convinced myself that my deplorable situation was somehow acceptable. It became my new reality. The alcohol had even changed my perception of this awful reality.

Soon, the utilities were shut off, and I thought, *Do I really need power? I have alcohol; that's all I need.* Then the water was turned off, and I thought, *Water isn't essential. I can shower at the community center when necessary. As long as I have my alcohol.* Eventually, they changed the locks on my home, seizing my home and all my belongings. The sheriff permitted me to retrieve a few personal items, but I declined. Not even photographs of my children held value. I chose instead to take only a few bottles of alcohol that remained in the house, promising myself that I would return for the rest later. I never did.

Do I really need a home? I questioned. *I still have a car. I can sleep there or find a cheap hotel. I have my alcohol. I'll manage somehow.* In the depths of my addiction, each acceptable new low became tolerable as long as I had my drugs and alcohol. My distorted perception embraced this new, distorted reality.

I relocated to a modest condominium, until that, too, slipped through my fingers with an eviction. Eventually, my car was repossessed. I borrowed a truck from a friend and sought refuge in a shabby hotel room conveniently close to a liquor store. I was convinced that everything would work out. I had enough money for alcohol, so I could manage. At least, that's what I told myself.

What I expected to be a temporary situation stretched into eighteen months. Every day, I would traverse the distance between my hotel and the liquor store on foot, scraping together the necessary funds. The routine became ingrained: beg, borrow, and scrape by each day, forsaking meals and drowning myself in alcohol. During that year, I believed I had reached rock bottom. But I hadn't even come close.

A year later, I found myself facing back-to-back DUI arrests, one of which involved wrecking my friend's truck, which he promptly took back from me. I became homeless. No car, no home, no money—just a lost soul wandering the streets of Salt Lake City. I survived in seedy hotel rooms or anywhere else I could find solace and indulge in alcohol around the clock. My children had given up on me, convinced that I had a death wish and would drink myself into oblivion. Many days, I questioned if I had finally reached rock bottom. But I hadn't even scratched the surface. Just an acceptable new low.

Over the next year, alcohol became my sole sustenance. My memory of that period is hazy at best. My days blurred together, consumed by fear and anxiety about acquiring enough money for alcohol and a place to sleep. I no longer feared my own demise or the rejection of the world; my only fear was not having enough money to fuel my addiction throughout the day and night.

My daily routine revolved around consuming at least one-fifth of vodka in the morning, followed by another at night to facilitate sleep before waking up, usually around three a.m., to finish whatever alcohol remained, ensuring

I could go back to sleep and repeat the cycle anew. Each day, I would embark on a long walk between liquor stores, masking my intoxication to avoid being denied a sale. This routine began after a liquor store manager refused to serve me due to my inebriation.

Little did I realize that I had not yet experienced the true depths of my addiction.

To sustain my alcohol consumption and the nineteen dollars required for the dilapidated hotel room infested with roaches, I resorted to extreme measures. For a significant portion of that year, I found myself panhandling on street corners near my temporary abode. Holding a sign that read, "Please Help! VETERAN Needs Your Help!" scrawled in black marker on a piece of cardboard, I sought donations from passersby. When the funds were insufficient for the hotel, I resigned myself to sleeping outdoors, ensuring that alcohol remained within my grasp. I grew out my beard, donned a hat and tattered clothes to avoid recognition.

I distinctly recall the horror I felt one day when a former business associate, accompanied by his wife and children, stopped their car beside me, rolled down the window, and handed me five dollars. I was convinced they had recognized me, yet I quickly realized they hadn't. I surmised that my disguise must be effective. Unbeknownst to my distorted mind, I had withered away from my usual weight of 190 pounds to a mere 140 pounds, unkempt, unwashed, and clad in tattered attire. Another acceptable low.

During this time, I discovered that panhandling often yielded just enough for the hotel room and an additional $9.85. This extra amount was precisely what I needed for a fifth-sized bottle of the cheapest vodka available, which I would then obtain from the liquor store. If I ran out of alcohol during the day, I would repeat the cycle. At times, I would think to myself, "Surely, this must be the lowest point I've reached." But I was far from the bottom. An acceptable new low.

Anger consumed me—anger toward the world, toward God, and most of all, toward myself. I felt cornered, desperate, and determined not to seek help from anyone, no matter the circumstances. I was convinced that no one cared.

Christmas that year, without a shred of doubt, stands as one of the most arduous trials I have ever been through. The significance of Christmas in my life had always been monumental, a cherished cornerstone of my existence. The joy of doting upon my beloved children, crafting moments of bliss, was a privilege I held dear. Fate had woven a different tapestry this year, a tapestry marred by my own undoing.

The clutches of my unruly drinking, more savage and untamed than ever, had transformed me into a mere vessel of a man, drifting aimlessly through days shrouded in a haze of perpetual blackout. In the abyss of my existence,

I found myself alone, homeless, and scraping by within the confines of a meager, threadbare hotel room. Aware of the dangerous nature of my affliction, my own mother, wise beyond measure, withheld any form of monetary aid, knowing all too well that it would only fuel the fire that consumed me.

However, in a final flicker of hope, she helped me salvage a semblance of Christmas spirit, not for myself, but for my children. She entrusted me with the use of a department store credit card, which happened to be across the way from my hotel. She also picked up a cheap cell phone so that I could connect with my children at Christmas. It was a modest gesture, a feeble attempt to rekindle flickering flames of joy. With the fragile card clutched tightly, I ventured out to procure meager offerings for my precious children. In the face of their modesty, it was but a droplet in an ocean of desires, yet it brought me a fleeting serenity, a momentary break from the suffocating grip of despair.

Driven by a desperate longing to connect, I reached out, leaving messages and texts, blindly hoping for a reunion during the holiday season. It had not dawned upon me, clouded by my own anguish, that they sought refuge from the demon that ravaged my mind and body.

As the eve of Christmas descended, an insurmountable weight of desolation crushed my spirit. The poignant images of my beloved children nestled within the bosom of a loving family while I languished alone in the depths of a desolate hotel room, drowning my sorrows in an elixir of intoxication to numb the searing ache that gnawed at my very core.

And then, a glimmer pierced the shroud of darkness. A call, fragile yet laden with an opportunity for redemption, beckoned me. It was my daughter, extending an invitation to share a moment, a respite from my despair. With newfound hope pulsating through my veins, I hastily gathered their gifts, trembling, sick from alcohol withdrawal, praying for salvation.

As we headed to the movie theater, there was a glimmer of hope that we could find some unity amidst the chaos. But my sorry state betrayed me, casting a shadow of discomfort over our fragile reunion. Even beneath their forced smiles, it was clear that my drunkenness and illness burdened their tender hearts. With the exchange of gifts and a heavy silence, my daughter bid me farewell, leaving my shattered dreams behind in that lonely hotel room.

In that moment, everything unraveled, and the symphony of emotional and physical agony echoed through the depths of my soul. I lay on the bed, curled up in a ball, tormented cries escaping my trembling lips. Anguished, I pleaded with a higher power, "Why, God? Why have you abandoned me? How much more must I bear?" Desperate to numb the overwhelming sorrow, I sought solace in the deceptive embrace of a half-gallon bottle filled to the brim with vodka. I surrendered to its alluring oblivion, allowing it to consume me.

During the dark night, I regained consciousness. I could hear the soft whispers of my dear friend and his wife as they sat on the edge of my bed.

Their words carried a sense of urgency, delivering a sobering truth. "Cord, you have to get up. Your life is at stake. You have to get up or you will die in this hotel room."

I closed my tired eyes, clinging to their voices as my lifeline. But as I opened my eyes once more, they had vanished, leaving behind only faint echoes, urging me to stop my self-destructive path. I realized I was hallucinating. I could not see them any longer, but their voices still continued, demanding that I stand up to do something about my own undoing and embark on a journey toward healing—a journey that held the key to my very survival.

As I lay their listening to their voices, I experienced a terrifying withdrawal episode, so severe that I believed I was on the brink of death. Desperate, I called my mother, a retired nurse, to explain what was happening. She urged me to seek hospitalization, warning that such a catastrophic withdrawal could trigger seizures, strokes, or heart attacks. Instead, I foolishly opted to drink more, hoping to quell the withdrawal symptoms while conversing with her. I consumed an entire bottle of vodka in a feeble attempt to alleviate my suffering, only to collapse on the floor. It was during that call that I had a violent seizure and heart failure, witnessed by my helpless mother on the other end of the line, who listened as I took my last breath and immediately dialed 911.

I awoke to the cacophony of emergency room personnel, doctors, and nurses scurrying around, diligently attending to their duties. A physician approached me and matter-of-factly explained that my heart had stopped, requiring the use of defibrillation paddles to revive me. He went on to explain to me that I was suffering from liver and kidney issues along with esophagus and severe internal bleeding. A crisis worker inquired about suicidal thoughts, to which I retorted, "Are you kidding me? Of course, I do! Can't you people just tell me how to end this?"

Surely, this must be the bottom, right? But I was still far from it. It was a new low that I was convinced I could still manage.

I spent a few days in ICU and then was admitted for nine days of detoxification. My physical condition worsened with each passing day. During this eventful stay, a doctor visited me. In a calm, matter-of-fact manner, he delivered a grave diagnosis.

"Mr. Beatty," he began, "you have alcoholic hepatitis and cirrhosis of the liver." Confused, I sought clarification. He explained, "Your liver has completely failed. An ultrasound revealed no functionality. We need to conduct a biopsy."

The results were devastating. My liver was beyond repair, and no liver transplant was available for someone in my condition. Additionally, I was informed that I suffered from esophagitis, experiencing internal bleeding, and my body was becoming septic. My kidneys were failing, and my heart palpitations foreshadowed an impending stroke or heart failure that was inevitably coming.

In desperation, I asked the doctor, "What can we do to fix this?"

His response pierced me to the core. "There is no fix, Cord. You have reached the point of no return. There is no liver transplant or hope for recovery. I advise you to settle your affairs, contact your children and loved ones, and we will do what we can to make you more comfortable."

"What am I supposed to do with this knowledge?" I pleaded with the desperation of a dying man.

He replied simply, "Pray," before briskly exiting the room.

Finally, I had found the unacceptable new low.

In that pivotal moment of my life, lying in the hospital bed, I was struck with a profound realization that my life on this earth had just ended.

The gravity of my drinking problem became undeniably clear.

As the next two days stretched on, I found myself engulfed in a sea of physical and emotional pain, consumed by anger and withdrawal. My fear of death turned to a fear of living another minute in this pain and suffering. The weight of my actions and the devastating impact on my loved children weighed heavily on my heart. I felt utterly defeated, broken, and overwhelmed by a deep desire to escape it all, even if it meant giving up on life itself. I couldn't fathom facing my children or family after what I had put them through. The shame and guilt gnawed at my soul.

Amidst the agony and sleepless nights, an unexpected visitor appeared in my hospital room. Whether it was a figment of my imagination, a dream, or something more, I can't say for certain. This mysterious figure exuded confidence and charm, captivating me with a charismatic presence. He posed uncomfortable questions about the immortality I sought, offering an alluring but sinister alternative solution. I grew increasingly uneasy as the conversation progressed, sensing that this individual was not what he seemed. He insidiously whispered that I had no one to turn to, that he was the only one left who loved me, and that he held all the answers and everything I desired. Discomfort turned to alarm, and I demanded his immediate departure.

"Okay, I'll be around," he responded, leaving a lingering sense of unease.

What happened next took me by surprise. Overwhelmed by pain and desperation, I tumbled off the bed and fell to my knees, crying out in a prayer that was more heartfelt and impassioned than anything I had ever uttered before. It was an outward expression of grief, a plea for forgiveness from my children, and a desperate call for divine intervention.

"Please, God, help me! Please, help me!" I beseeched, pouring out my anguish and surrendering to a force greater than myself.

I had reached the bottom. The unacceptable new low.

At that moment, I finally let go of my pride, ego, illusions of control, and delusional image of myself, my stubborn resistance. Defeated, alone, and stripped of all pretenses, I was at the mercy of my circumstances. Physically and emotionally drained, I pleaded with God, abandoning all resistance and declaring my willingness to be taken from this world. "I give up. Please, God, please take me. I can't bear to live another moment of this anguish. I don't know what you want from me. Just take me now!"

Exhausted and broken, I cried myself to sleep on the cold hospital floor.

When I awoke the next morning, my eyes met the gaze of a vibrant bluebird perched on the windowsill. In that moment, an inexplicable shift occurred. All the pain, anger, depression, anxiety, loneliness, and fear that had consumed me vanished. It was as if a divine presence had intervened, cradling me in a profound sense of love, peace, and serenity. The weight of my burdens had somehow been lifted, replaced by a newfound awareness that someone had gently guided me back to the bed during the night when I was too weak to stand.

I finally grasped the true meaning of powerlessness.

On this life-altering, unforgettable morning, God was doing for me what I could no longer do for myself. I recognized that my life had been devoid of a connection with God. I had been running away from him for so long, not understanding that his spiritual presence was what I desperately needed in my life. God held all the power, and I, in my surrender, finally accepted my own powerlessness.

Four days later, against the advice of medical professionals, I mustered the strength to leave the hospital. I reached out to my mother, humbly asking if I could seek refuge in her home for a while, yearning for a haven to embark on my healing journey. From the moment I awakened that morning in that hospital room, I felt a palpable presence of God surrounding me. A profound sense of peace enveloped my being, and I knew deep in my soul that this was the turning point, the beginning of a transformative journey toward a life of sobriety.

In the days that followed, I embarked on a path of recovery unlike anything I had ever experienced. Every step I took was guided by a newfound faith and an unwavering trust in a power greater than myself and the unmistakable conviction of my own powerlessness. I immersed myself in prayer and meditation, seeking solace and guidance in the divine. It was the strength and resilience I needed to confront the challenges ahead.

As I settled into my mother's home, I embraced the healing process with a renewed determination. I was very sick and knew that I had a long way to go. I surrounded myself with a supportive network of loved ones who understood the gravity of my journey and stood by my side unconditionally. Together, we created a space of understanding, compassion, and accountability—a sanctuary where I could share my fears, insecurities, and triumphs.

Each day became a testament to my commitment to sobriety. I no longer relied on self-medication to drown out the pain or escape the reality of my past. Instead, I confronted my demons head-on, working through the deep-rooted issues that fueled my addiction. With the support of a mentor and the guidance of recovery programs, I delved into the Twelve Steps, examining my shortcomings and making amends to those that I had harmed.

It was during this transformative process that I realized the true meaning of acceptance and surrender. It wasn't a sign of weakness but rather an act of courage—a conscious choice to relinquish control and place my faith in something greater than myself. I acknowledged my powerlessness over alcohol and embraced the notion that my journey to lasting recovery required a spiritual awakening.

With a newfound sense of humility, I opened myself to the possibility of change.

In my daily practice of prayer and meditation, I discovered a profound connection to the divine. My every waking moment was filled with constant communication with my creator. I found solace in surrendering my worries, fears, and desires, trusting that I was being guided along the path of recovery. It was through this spiritual connection that I began to experience a sense of serenity and purpose, replacing the void that alcohol had once filled.

With time, the wounds of the past started to heal, and I embarked on the process of rebuilding my life. I mended broken relationships, making amends to those I had harmed and working diligently to rebuild trust. I sought professional help to address the underlying issues that contributed to my addiction, attending therapy sessions and participating in support groups to gain valuable insights and coping mechanisms.

As the days turned into weeks and the weeks into months, I witnessed a profound transformation taking place within me. I no longer identified as a victim of addiction but as a survivor, armed with newfound resilience and a deep sense of self-awareness.

The journey was not without its challenges—temptations and triggers lurked in unexpected places—but with a solid support system and an unwavering commitment to my sobriety, I navigated these obstacles with grace and perseverance.

Today, I stand as a testament to the power of surrender and the transformative nature of recovery. My experience serves as a reminder that hitting rock bottom was not the end but rather the catalyst for a profound spiritual awakening and a life filled with purpose and meaning. By surrendering my will to a higher power, I discovered a strength within myself that I never knew existed—a strength that continues to guide me on the path of sobriety, serenity, peace, and freedom.

These personal experiences provided me with a glimmer of newfound hope and desire to share my story.

Allow me to illuminate the path before us as we look at Step Two of this transformative journey together.

Step Two demands honesty from us. It demands that we first have profound and life-changing Step One. A fully conceding moment of clarity concerning our powerlessness.

Step Two reads: "I came to believe that a power greater than I could restore my sanity."

The authors of the book of Alcoholics Anonymous expressed, "Once I can acknowledge the potential existence of a higher power or God, I will be enveloped by an unprecedented sensation of strength and guidance—one that surpasses any previous encounters, as long as I remain open to taking the remaining eleven steps."

Observe how the authors emphasize the word "new." They do not refer to something from the past or a familiar experience you might have had before. Instead, they speak of a fresh encounter that awaits you, ready to be embraced and received. This signifies a new path unfolding before you, accompanied by a power unlike any you have ever known. It implies discovering a direction you have never ventured upon. This is what lies ahead—something we can eagerly anticipate.

Before concluding Step One, I encourage you to reflect on the meaning of "powerless" once more.

At my treatment centers, many individuals arrive in a state of denial, reluctant to acknowledge the existence of a power greater than themselves. A significant number of them hold the belief that there is no God. Typically, I address this matter swiftly.

Allow me to pose a question: Have you ever found yourself curled up in a fetal position on your bed, overwhelmed by extreme depression, anxiety, pain, misery, despair, and desperation? Have you experienced a sense of brokenness, loneliness, defeat, and hopelessness that you found devastatingly overwhelming? In that vulnerable state, have you clasped your hands tightly to your face, softly pleading out loud, "Please help me"?

Now, let me ask you: To whom were you directing those words? Every man, woman, and child is born with a fundamental inner knowing of a power greater than ourselves. For some of us, it takes getting to that unacceptable new low where we find the desperation of a dying man to remember it. In the military they used to say, "There are no atheists in a foxhole." This is a true statement.

Ask yourself, "Is my life currently manageable, or has it devolved into the chaotic and confusing three-ring circus discussed earlier?"

Ask yourself, "Can I wholeheartedly admit to my deepest self that I lack the power to resolve my problems independently?"

CHAPTER 5

UNDERSTANDING POWERLESSNESS. A SPIRITUAL JOURNEY

The story of my journey to sobriety is a tapestry woven with paradoxes, shaping my understanding of powerlessness. It all began with a profound realization that completely transformed my life—I discovered that I was truly powerless. I experienced the desperation of a dying man, reaching the bottom of my addiction. No longer could I manage or control my disease; all I had left was sheer desperation. It was in this place of surrender, where I conceded to my powerlessness and opened myself to something greater, that my path to recovery began.

There were two distinct paths that converged and led me to a deeper understanding of myself. One was a program that taught me to acknowledge my powerlessness over addiction. The other was the enlightening interpretations of ancient wisdom found in the teachings of respected authors.

In the midst of my recovery from addiction and mental illness, I felt like I was constantly battling against a relentless current, struggling to stay afloat. Always seeking an answer, going to a meeting every day and asking God to keep me sober for just one more day. During this time, I studied the teachings of Alcoholics Anonymous, *The Secret*,

Wayne Dwyer's *Change Your Thoughts Change Your Life, Tao Te Ching* by Lao-Tzu, and many others. It was during this struggle that I stumbled upon a book, where insightful interpretations of ancient wisdom resonated with me deeply. The emphasis on surrendering and letting go as pathways to freedom caught my attention and began to shape my thoughts and direction.

One particular concept spoke to me—the principle of "effortless action" or "action through inaction." It spoke to me about aligning myself with the natural flow of life rather than resisting it. It meant surrendering to the order of things and recognizing and accepting our human limitations.

In my battle with addiction, I fought against the constant mental obsession. Every day was an exhausting struggle, leaving me feeling defeated. I was in a perpetual state of resistance, unable to understand why I couldn't simply break free.

My addiction was like a relentless storm, with dark clouds of desire swirling in my mind. The cravings were like strong winds, pushing and pulling me in unpredictable directions. I tried to shield myself from the storm, desperately clinging to the hope of sobriety, but the storm's power was overwhelming. Each day felt like an uphill battle, and each night I silently prayed for relief.

My mind was trapped in a loop, repeating the same thoughts over and over again. These were the lies I told myself, the anthem of my addiction. Their deafening chorus drowned out the faint voice that pleaded for help and change.

Resistance became my constant companion. I waged a civil war within the confines of my own mind, stubbornly refusing to surrender to the enemy—my addiction. I was lost on a battlefield of my own making, my life spiraling out of control, and my soul burdened with despair.

I questioned my strength and willpower, blaming myself for being weak and unable to quit. It was a cycle of guilt, shame, and disappointment, spinning faster with each passing day. Yet, I was trapped in the endless loop of addiction, unable to break free.

Then, a thought struck me—what if, instead of struggling against my addiction, I embraced it? What if I accepted my powerlessness and stopped fighting the current? This shift in perspective was revolutionary for me. For the first time, I realized that I wasn't succumbing to cravings but battling a disease.

Acknowledging powerlessness was not about accepting defeat; it was about surrendering to the reality of my situation. It meant letting go of the illusion of control and aligning myself with the natural flow of life. It required recognizing my human limitations and understanding that the power to overcome addiction didn't lie in resistance but in acceptance and surrender.

I found myself entangled in the shadows of addiction and self-defeat, lost in a dense fog of despair. It was during this time that I stumbled upon a ray of wisdom that changed the course of my journey.

As I share this journey with you, dear reader, I invite you to join me in introspection. Pause and ask yourself the questions I pose along the way, for within them, you might just find your own answers.

Do you remember a time when you felt utterly powerless? When you have found yourself trapped in a destructive cycle, repeating the same mistakes over and over again? I remember that feeling all too well. In the depths of my addiction, I believed I was in control of my fate, the captain of my soul. But the reality was far from it.

That's when I stumbled upon the teachings of respected authors. Their interpretation of powerlessness was both unfamiliar and intriguing. They spoke about ancient wisdom, drawing upon the timeless principles of spirituality. In aligning these teachings with the idea of surrendering to powerlessness, I began to see it not as a weakness but as a surrender. Can you imagine that? Transforming something that feels inherently negative into a positive force of change?

These teachings guide us to flow like water, to surrender to our path, and to accept our human limitations. Can you embrace the idea of relinquishing the illusion of control and moving in harmony with the natural rhythm of life?

In admitting my powerlessness over addiction, I discovered an inexplicable strength. Paradoxically, by acknowledging my weakness, I gained newfound power. It was a paradox that defied conventional understanding, but it was undeniably real.

These teachings, in their infinite wisdom, reinforced the concept of surrender. They taught me that life, like a river, follows its own course. We can either swim against the current, exhausting ourselves in the process, or we can surrender and allow the river to carry us along. Can you visualize the act of surrender, not as a defeat an aligning with the greater flow of life?

My journey was one of understanding, recovery, and self-discovery. And it all began with acknowledging my powerlessness, embracing the wisdom of respected authors, and taking that first step toward change.

As you reflect on this, ask yourself: What does powerlessness mean to you? Are you willing to surrender to the flow of life, to accept your human limitations? Are you ready to embark on your own journey of recovery, taking that crucial first step? Remember, every journey starts with a single step. Are you ready to take yours?

As I delved deeper into my journey of self-discovery, I began to realize that powerlessness wasn't a destination; it was a guidepost. It served as a steppingstone on the path to self-awareness. Now, as you read these words, I encourage you to ponder: Have you recognized your own guideposts?

Can you see the steppingstones that could lead you to your own recovery?

In surrendering to the flow, I found a sense of peace I had never experienced before. Instead of battling against the current of life, I began to swim with it. Instead of being overpowered by my addiction, I chose to release my illusion of control over it. It was a subtle yet profound shift. Can you envision such a transformation in your own life?

Of course, there were still hurdles to overcome. Accepting powerlessness didn't mean eradicating challenges or avoiding discomfort in my life. Instead, it meant changing my relationship with those challenges. Rather than seeing them as insurmountable obstacles, I started viewing them as opportunities for growth. This shift in perspective, inspired by the teachings of respected authors, had a significant impact on my journey. Can you find a way to reinterpret the challenges you face in your own life?

As I progressed on this path, I discovered that surrendering didn't leave me feeling helpless, as I initially feared. On the contrary, it granted me strength and resilience, empowering me to move forward with grace and patience.

Can you imagine the liberation that comes from relinquishing the need to control every aspect of your life? Can you grasp the empowerment that stems from surrendering to the ebb and flow of the universe?

My journey wasn't without its struggles, but it was transformative. And it all began with that crucial first step—the admission of powerlessness. Your journey, too, will be unique and challenging, but remember that every step you take brings you closer to a new and healthier version of yourself.

So, I ask you again: Are you ready to acknowledge your own powerlessness? Are you prepared to surrender to your human limitations and, in doing so, open the door to growth, healing, and self-discovery? Are you ready to take that first step?

As I continued to align myself with these spiritual teachings and principles, my perspective began to shift. I started to view my struggles not as failures but as opportunities for learning and personal growth. Can you see your own struggles through this lens? Are you willing to view your setbacks as chances to gain deeper insights into yourself, your strengths, and your weaknesses?

I vividly remember the realization that hit me: By admitting my powerlessness over addiction, I wasn't expressing weakness. Instead, I was acknowledging the courage it takes to confront the reality of my situation. Does it seem counterintuitive to you? The idea that admitting powerlessness can be a display of strength?

These authors often spoke of the beauty of paradox, and it was within this paradox that I discovered my empowerment. Surrendering to my own human limitations set me free. It allowed me to accept that I couldn't control everything, especially my addiction. This surrender, however, wasn't a sign of defeat. It was an admission that I am human, prone to making mistakes and experiencing shortcomings—and that was okay. Have you ever found comfort in such paradoxes? Can you see the power that comes from admitting your vulnerabilities and limitations?

As I continued to surrender, I found myself becoming more attuned to my own needs and emotions. I navigated my journey of recovery with greater understanding and patience for myself. This wasn't something I achieved overnight; it was an ongoing process, with each day bringing new lessons and challenges. Can you relate to this in your own life? Have you discovered that each day brings its own unique set of challenges and lessons?

Through acknowledging my powerlessness and embracing these teachings, I uncovered a new form of power—the power of self-awareness, self-acceptance, and self-love. This power doesn't seek to control or dominate; instead, it nurtures and empowers. It stems from truly knowing oneself and accepting oneself, flaws and all. Can you see how this power can support you on your journey to recovery? Are you willing to explore the potential within yourself?

So, as we continue walking this path together, I encourage you to consider these questions. Are you ready to surrender to your own human limitations and acknowledge your powerlessness? Are you prepared to find strength in vulnerability and empowerment in surrender? Because that is where our journey to recovery truly begins.

On this transformative journey, spirituality plays a vital role. It's not about subscribing to a specific religion or worshiping a particular deity; rather, it's about connecting with a power greater than ourselves—a higher force that can guide us on the path to recovery. Have you ever experienced a deep sense of connection with a higher power? Can you open yourself up to the possibility of such a connection?

This is where the spiritual teachings and principles come into play. They represent the true nature of the world and the guiding force of the universe. They embody the principles of flow, balance, and the interconnectedness of all things. Can you imagine aligning yourself with this flow, allowing it to guide your thoughts and actions?

Let's consider water, a powerful symbol in Taoist philosophy. It possesses a softness and a yielding nature, yet over time, it can shape even the hardest of rocks. It effortlessly navigates around obstacles in its path, always finding a way forward. It doesn't strive or struggle; it simply is. Can you see the potential in becoming like water, in yielding to the flow of life rather than resisting it?

In recognizing our powerlessness over addiction, we are taking the first step toward becoming like water. We acknowledge that trying to break through the rock of addiction with force and resistance is futile. Instead, we seek a different path. It's not about fighting against the current but about learning to move with it. Can you see how this might apply to your own life and struggles?

These authors often emphasized the importance of aligning our personal will with the divine will, surrendering our ego-driven desires to the guidance of a higher power. This isn't about giving up or relinquishing control; it's about aligning ourselves with the universal flow of energy. By doing so, we allow the universe to guide us and help us navigate the challenges of addiction and recovery. Can you surrender your will to this higher power, allowing it to illuminate your path to recovery?

In acknowledging our powerlessness, we tap into a much greater source of power. We embrace the paradox of powerlessness and invite the spiritual principles to guide us on our journey. It's a transformative process, a path that leads us toward self-discovery, healing, and growth, because that, my friends, is where true recovery begins.

The first step of the recovery journey brings spiritual exploration into focus. It is the moment we humbly acknowledge our need for guidance. It is the point where we open ourselves to the idea of a higher power, which forms the foundation for the subsequent steps.

Take a moment to reflect: Have you ever felt a connection with something larger than yourself? It could have been a moment of awe while gazing at the night sky, a moment of peace in the presence of nature, or a moment of profound love and connection with another person. These experiences provide glimpses of the higher power that is central to the recovery journey.

When we admit powerlessness over addiction, we create space in our lives. Initially, this space may feel unsettling, filled with loss and uncertainty. However, it also becomes a gateway to a new kind of power—a spiritual power. The remaining steps guide us through this gateway, exploring and defining our understanding of a higher power, establishing a connection with it, and surrendering our will and lives to its guidance. As we go further into this journey, we embark on a path of seeking, discovering, and deepening our relationship with a higher power that resonates with our hearts and aligns with our values.

Through surrender, we tap into a wellspring of strength and resilience that comes from aligning ourselves with the universal flow of energy. We no longer need to rely solely on our own limited resources; instead, we draw upon the infinite wisdom of the higher power.

In this surrender, we find freedom. It is not a surrender of defeat but rather an act of empowerment. By recognizing our limitations and acknowledging that there is a force greater than ourselves, we release the burden of trying to control every aspect of our lives. We learn to trust in the unfolding of a greater plan and to navigate our recovery journey with humility, openness, and faith.

The spiritual teachings and principles we encounter along this path provide us with tools and perspectives to support our recovery. They teach us to embrace the paradoxes of life, to find strength in vulnerability, and to cultivate resilience through surrender. They guide us to let go of our ego-driven desires and to align ourselves with a higher purpose that goes beyond our individual selves.

As we walk this spiritual journey, we may encounter moments of deep connection, profound insights, and transformative experiences. We learn to listen to our inner wisdom, to trust our intuition, and to recognize the signs and synchronicities that guide us along the way.

It's important to remember that spirituality is a personal and ever-evolving aspect of our recovery. Each individual's journey is unique, and there is no right or wrong way to explore and embrace spirituality. What matters is the willingness to open ourselves up to the possibility of a higher power, to surrender our will and lives to its guidance, and to cultivate a sense of connection and purpose that supports our healing and growth.

So, as you continue on your own spiritual journey of recovery, I encourage you to remain open-minded and curious. Allow the teachings and principles to speak to you in their own way, and trust in your own inner guidance as you navigate this transformative path. Remember that true power lies in surrender and that by embracing your powerlessness, you open yourself up to a world of possibility and transformation.

You may face challenges and setbacks along the way, but know that they are part of your growth and learning. Embrace them as opportunities for self-reflection and resilience. Stay committed to your recovery, and know that the power to heal and transform resides within you.

As you embark on this spiritual journey, surround yourself with a supportive community that understands and shares your commitment to recovery. Seek out mentors, teachers, or fellow seekers who can guide and inspire you along the way. Share your experiences, struggles, and triumphs with others who can provide understanding and encouragement.

Remember, your recovery journey is not a solitary one. It is a collective effort that involves both your own inner work and the support of others. Together, we can overcome the challenges of addiction, find healing, and embrace a life of purpose and fulfillment.

So, my friend, are you ready to take that leap of faith and embark on a spiritual journey of recovery? Are you ready to surrender to a power greater than yourself, to release the illusion of control, and to align with the universal flow of energy? If so, trust in yourself and trust in the journey that awaits you. It may not always be easy, but it will be worth it. Step by step, surrender by surrender, you will discover the strength, wisdom, and freedom that lie within you.

CHAPTER 6

UNDERSTANDING THE POWER OF SPIRITUAL SURRENDER

The spiritual surrender may be the most difficult part of Step One. Stepping outside our ourselves to rely on a higher power doesn't come easy.

In the turmoil of my own struggle, I came face to face with a truth that changed my life: the notion of spiritual surrender. To a military veteran, the term 'surrender' always brings up thoughts of defeat or loss for me, but in the context of spirituality and personal growth, it took on a profoundly different meaning.

Spiritual surrender is about releasing the illusion of control we think we have over our lives and trusting in a higher power; however, you choose to define that. It is a conscious decision to turn over our will, and our life, to the care of this greater force. This might sound like a loss of personal agency, but it is quite the opposite.

Spiritual surrender is not a passive act. It is not about giving up or relinquishing responsibility for our actions. Rather, it is an active and deliberate choice to align ourselves with the flow of life, with the belief that there is a higher power at work that wants the best for us. It is about humility, yes, but it is also about faith. It is the ultimate act of trust, a leap of faith into the unknown, the belief that even if we cannot see the entire path laid out before us, we are being guided in the right direction.

Are you tired of fighting against the current of your life, trying to swim upstream against the flow? Do you feel like you're holding onto the reins of your life so tightly your hands are cramping and your knuckles are white? Have you considered that there might be a different way, a path of less resistance and more peace? Are you willing to consider the possibility that letting go, surrendering your struggles, and trusting in a force greater than yourself could lead you to a life of greater peace, purpose, and fulfillment?

Let me assure you that spiritual surrender does not equate to weakness or defeat. It is a powerful choice that takes tremendous courage. It is a journey of faith and trust, a dance with the divine. It requires us to let go of our ego-driven need to control and to embrace uncertainty, knowing that we are guided and held. It was only when I fully embraced the concept of spiritual surrender that I was able to break the chains of my addiction.

Through surrender, I allowed divine intervention to enter my life. I stopped fighting and started listening. I opened myself up to the wisdom of a higher power and allowed it to guide me. And as I did, I found a strength I never knew I had. It was not the aggressive, resistant strength I had been clinging to before but a gentle, resilient power that rose from my willingness to trust and let go. And I am here to tell you that it is a journey worth taking.

It is a journey of liberation, a journey home to the true essence of who you are.

In surrendering, I found myself better able to handle the challenges of my addiction. I replaced my desperation and despair with faith and acceptance. I stopped trying to dictate how my recovery should look and instead trusted the process laid out for me in the Twelve Steps.

Are you familiar with the saying, "Let go and let God"? You hear it a lot in meetings of AA or NA. Let go and let God. What does that even mean?

This saying encapsulates the essence of spiritual surrender. It's the acknowledgement that we are not the ultimate authorities in our lives. It doesn't mean that we stop doing the necessary work or become passive in our recovery. Instead, it means we trust that when we take right action, the results will take care of themselves, according to a plan greater than our own.

For me, the concept of letting go and spiritually surrendering to a higher power was a welcome beacon of light shining brightly. Especially for someone with the desperation of a dying man.

For me, the act of surrender came with a wave of relief. Have you ever tried to control every aspect of your life down to the minutest detail? It's exhausting, isn't it? The truth is, the more I tried to control, the more out of control I felt. But surrendering that need to control released a huge burden off my shoulders. I could breathe. I could focus on what I could do and let go of what was out of my hands.

I know that admitting powerlessness can be scary. It was for me too. We're so used to equating powerlessness with helplessness. But the first step of AA does not ask us to become helpless. It asks us to acknowledge that our lives had become unmanageable and that we were powerless over alcohol. It doesn't mean that we are powerless over our recovery or our future.

So, I pose these questions to you: Are you tired of fighting a battle you can't win on your own? Are you ready to let go of your need to control? Are you willing to trust in a power greater than yourself? Can you find the courage to surrender, knowing that in doing so, you're opening yourself up to divine guidance and unlimited potential for change and growth?

Surrender is an act of faith and humility, of admitting our human limitations and opening ourselves up to the divine. It is not about giving up but about allowing something greater than ourselves to guide our journey. It's about trust, hope, and acceptance. It's about opening the door to a life beyond what we can see or control. Spiritual surrender was my turning point, and it could be yours too. Are you ready to take that step?

It's important to recognize that spiritual surrender doesn't mean we don't take responsibility for our actions. We still do the work. We still make amends. We still strive for progress in our recovery. What it means is that we acknowledge that we aren't alone in this journey and that a higher power can guide us along this path.

This journey isn't just about freeing ourselves from the shackles of addiction or mental illness. It's about growing, evolving, and becoming the best versions of ourselves that we can be. I remember when I was going through the Twelve Steps and I truly realized this. Do you realize that your journey doesn't end with sobriety? Do you understand that sobriety is just the first step toward self-improvement and growth?

This is the beauty of surrender. It's not a passive act but an active process of releasing, accepting, and trusting. It's a paradigm shift from a mindset of struggle and resistance to one of acceptance and flow. It's about recognizing our human limitations but not allowing them to limit us.

Remember, powerlessness doesn't mean weakness. It doesn't mean that we're devoid of strength, will, or ability. It simply means that we are human. And in our humanity, in our imperfection, we find our greatest strength. For it is when we admit that we can't do this alone that we open ourselves to the power of something greater, something divine.

Are you ready to let go and let God? Are you ready to find power in your powerlessness? It is a journey, a process, but trust me when I say it is a journey worth embarking upon.

As we move forward, I want to assure you that each step is just as crucial as the last. Each serves a purpose, and every step you take on this journey brings you one step closer to the strength, clarity, and peace you deserve.

One might wonder, *Why is surrendering my will and my life over to the care of a God or Higher Power so crucial to my recovery?* Well, that's where faith comes in. When we place our faith in a Higher Power, we make room for divine intervention to work in our lives. This faith is not just about believing in something greater than ourselves, it's about trusting this Higher Power to guide us on our journey to recovery and self-discovery. Can you see the shift? The shift from living in fear to living in faith? The shift from struggling to control to surrendering control and trusting the process?

When you move to Step Two, which is coming to believe that a power greater than ourselves could restore us to sanity, you're opening yourself up to the idea of faith. To trust that something outside of yourself can help restore you to a state of peace and wholeness.

And then there's Step Three. This is where you make the decision to turn your will and your life over to the care of this Higher Power. This step can be challenging. It requires a deep level of trust and surrender. It requires you to let go of control, a thing many of us cling to, especially when our lives have felt so out of control due to addiction. But in this surrender, there's immense freedom.

This is not a journey you're expected to walk alone. That's why the steps and support groups exist; to guide you, to walk with you. It's about community, shared experience, empathy, and unconditional support.

As you navigate through your journey, remember this, surrender isn't about giving up, it's about giving in. Giving in to the fact that we can't control everything, but we can control our actions, our decisions, and our responses. And most importantly, it's about giving in to hope, faith, and a life that's worth living. How can you start practicing surrender in your life today?

When we make that leap of faith, when we surrender and give control over to our Higher Power, it changes our perspective on everything. Suddenly, we're not alone in this journey. We have a divine ally on our side, guiding us and providing us with the strength we need to overcome our challenges. This Higher Power, however, you choose to understand it, becomes a source of immense support and comfort. You're no longer battling addiction on your own but together with this greater presence.

This change in perspective brings about a significant transformation in how we approach our recovery process. It's no longer just about stopping the act of drinking or using drugs. It's about a holistic change, a complete transformation of mind, body, and spirit. This is why the Twelve Steps don't end with the cessation of the addictive behavior; they continue on to Steps Four through Twelve, which focus on personal growth, making amends, improving our conscious contact with our Higher Power, and carrying the message of recovery to others.

These steps guide us through an introspective journey where we examine our past mistakes, make amends where possible, and learn to live a life of humility, gratitude, and service to others. Can you see the potential for growth and transformation in these steps?

When we reach Step Twelve, having had a spiritual awakening as the result of these steps, we're asked to carry this message to other alcoholics and to practice these principles in all our affairs. This is the culmination of our journey, where we use our experiences and our recovery to help others. It's about paying it forward, about making a positive impact on the world. It is this final step that truly embodies the transformation that has occurred within us.

This surrender, this leap of faith into the unknown, is nothing short of terrifying. Yet it is in this fear where you might discover your most profound courage. Isn't it empowering to consider that in recognizing your powerlessness, you are making the first step toward regaining control of your life?

When you surrender, you're not waving a white flag of defeat. You're raising a banner of faith and hope. Faith in your Higher Power, whatever that may be, and hope in a brighter, sober future. You're choosing to step out of the endless cycle of addiction, out of isolation and into a community that understands your struggle and will be there to support you every step of the way. Can you feel that? That sense of community, of not being alone in this journey?

Each day is a new opportunity to reaffirm your commitment to your sobriety and your recovery. Have you ever had a moment in your life where you have had to choose to let go of control? What did it feel like? Was it frightening, liberating, or maybe a mix of both?

In the context of the Twelve Steps, this daily practice of surrender is what helps us establish and strengthen our connection with our Higher Power. The more we practice, the more we lean on this divine source of strength, the deeper and more meaningful our relationship becomes. Can you imagine the peace and comfort that comes from knowing that you're not alone, that you have a divine ally in your corner, supporting you, guiding you, providing you with strength and courage when you need it most?

Remember, the journey of a thousand miles begins with a single step. Your first step in this journey of recovery is admitting that you are powerless over your addiction and that your life has become unmanageable. But this admission is not a sign of defeat. It's a declaration of hope and faith. It's the starting point of your journey toward recovery, transformation, and spiritual growth. Are you ready to take that step?

CHAPTER 7

THE ROLE OF EGO IN POWERLESSNESS

The human ego is a complex and powerful force. It is our sense of self, our personal identity, and it plays a significant role in how we perceive the world and ourselves. One of the primary functions of the ego is to maintain our sense of control and independence. It does not like to admit defeat or vulnerability. Hence, the ego can become a significant obstacle in acknowledging our powerlessness, particularly in the context of addiction.

You see, the ego thrives on control. It wants to believe that it can handle everything, that it is invincible and untouchable. The idea of being powerless over anything, especially something as personal and consuming as addiction, is threatening to the ego. The ego wants to believe that we can stop whenever we want, that we just don't want to right now. It keeps us in a state of denial about the severity of our problem.

Why? Because acknowledging powerlessness means admitting that we're not in control. It means accepting that there's an aspect of our lives—our addiction—that we can't manage on our own. And for the ego, that's a tough pill to swallow.

Now, let's talk about pride, another facet of the ego.

Pride can make us refuse to admit that we have a problem. It tells us that admitting to having an addiction is a sign of weakness, that we're failures.

Admitting that we have an issue with addiction isn't a character flaw; it's an act of courage and honesty. Pride, a facet of our ego, can often stand as a roadblock on our path toward recovery and empowerment. It whispers to us that acknowledging our struggles with addiction is an admission of failure, a sign of weakness, a declaration of our inadequacy. This insidious voice can prevent us from seeking the help we need, trapping us in a cycle of denial and self-destruction.

But let's dispel this harmful misconception. There's a monumental difference between 'having a problem' and 'being a problem.' Everyone, regardless of their status, strength, or resilience, faces problems. Problems are external to us—they do not define our inherent worth or value. They are circumstances to be confronted, challenges to be overcome, lessons to be learned. Having a problem, such as an addiction, is not an indictment of your character; instead, it's a part of your current human experience.

'Being a problem' implies that the issue resides within our core identity, suggesting that we are inherently flawed or defective. This perspective is not only damaging but also inherently untrue. Our struggles do not define us. They do not make us 'problems.' They are situations we're dealing with, not who we are.

When we muster the courage to say, "I have a problem with addiction," we're not admitting defeat. Quite the opposite—we're exhibiting bravery, honesty, and self-awareness, we're recognizing that we're currently in a battle, but we're not surrendering to the enemy; instead, we're preparing to fight. We're affirming that while we might be struggling right now, we refuse to be defined by these struggles. We're expressing our intention to change our circumstances, to seek help, to embark on the journey of recovery.

Admitting that we have an addiction isn't a character flaw; it's an act of bravery. It is an assertion of our determination to reclaim our lives from the clutches of addiction. It's an acknowledgment of our humanity, our vulnerability, and our innate capacity for change and growth.

As we move past our pride and acknowledge our problems, we empower ourselves to face them, to seek help, to begin healing. We step out of the shadow of denial and into the light of acceptance, opening the door to transformation, growth, and ultimate empowerment. This is the real strength, the true victory over our egos, and the first, most crucial step on our journey from powerlessness to empowerment.

Furthermore, the ego can trick us into believing we're unique in our struggles. It isolates us, convincing us that no one else could possibly understand what we're going through. It whispers that we are alone in our battle, which could not be further from the truth. Millions of people worldwide have faced addiction, fought it, and found paths to recovery.

There's a profound power in shared experiences and mutual support that the ego tries to hide from us. Have you ever noticed your ego resisting the idea of asking for help? Can you recall a time when pride kept you from admitting a mistake or a struggle?

This is why ego deflation is often a significant part of recovery programs. It's about learning to step back, take an honest look at our lives, and admit where we have lost control. It's about understanding that it's okay to ask for help and that acknowledging our powerlessness doesn't make us weak; it opens the door for us to seek the help we need.

But remember, while our egos can hinder us, they also have a role to play in our recovery. Our sense of self can be a source of resilience and determination, pushing us forward on our journey toward sobriety. The key is not to let our egos dominate us but to find a balanced, healthier relationship with them.

The ego can be a significant barrier in acknowledging our powerlessness over addiction, but with awareness, honesty, and willingness, we can overcome this obstacle and make the first step toward recovery. We need to deflate our ego, not destroy it. This action isn't about diminishing our worth but about recognizing our human limitations and the reality of our situation. Does this resonate with you? Can you see the role your ego plays in your relationship with addiction and recovery?

I recall the day I finally saw my ego for what it was; a façade, a shield I'd constructed to protect myself from the harsh truth—that I was powerless over my addiction. My ego, which I once believed was my closest ally, had been an impenetrable barrier standing in the way of my recovery. It was my ego that told me I was different, that my addiction was something I could control on my own without anyone's help. Oh, how mistaken I was.

My ego had been feeding me lies, false narratives of invincibility and independence. I was trapped in a cycle of denial, refusing to see the reality of my situation. I couldn't accept the idea that I was powerless, that my life was spiraling out of control due to my addiction.

I can see now that it was my ego that isolated me, convincing me that I was alone in my battle, that no one else could possibly understand my struggles. I can recall nights when I sat in the darkness, my heart heavy with the weight of loneliness, the voice of my ego whispering that I was unique in my struggles. Looking back, can you identify those moments when your ego isolated you? Can you see how it might have stood in the way of asking for help?

It was not until I truly started to deflate my ego that I was able to accept my powerlessness and seek help. I had to dismantle the fortress I had built around myself, brick by brick. This process was not easy; it was painful and humbling. But it was also liberating. I came to understand that acknowledging my powerlessness did not make me weak; on the contrary, it opened a door for change, for recovery.

Yet, I also learned that deflating my ego didn't mean obliterating my sense of self. It was about balance. I needed my ego to push me forward, to fuel my determination to recover. But I had to ensure it was no longer the dominant force in my life. Are you able to distinguish when your ego is guiding you versus when it may be misleading you? Can you identify a healthy balance?

Accepting my powerlessness over my addiction, surrendering my will, and admitting I needed help was the beginning of my journey toward recovery. It's an ongoing journey, a daily decision to reject the lies of my ego and embrace the truth of my human limitations. It's the realization that I am not alone in my struggle, that there is strength and hope in shared experiences.

Can you recognize the need for balance in your life? Are you ready to let go of the ego's dominance and admit your powerlessness to move forward in your journey? The power to change begins with surrendering the illusions that the ego provides and embracing our true, authentic selves.

Our ego will insist that it is stronger than the addiction, that it can fight off the cravings without any outside help. This ego-driven perspective creates a narrative of invincibility, a narrative where admitting powerlessness is synonymous with admitting weakness.

Yet, it is this very narrative that will lead you deeper into the abyss of addiction. The ego's insistence on maintaining control, despite clear evidence of its inability to do so, will only exacerbate our struggle. It will isolate us from potential sources of help, fostering a false sense of self-reliance. The ego can indeed be a formidable opponent on our path to recovery and empowerment. It often assumes the role of a deceptive storyteller, spinning narratives of invincibility and self-sufficiency that, while seemingly empowering, serve only to deepen our struggles.

One of the most pervasive stories it tells is that of self-reliance. In this narrative, our ego paints us as lone warriors, strong and capable enough to conquer addiction's powerful hold all by ourselves. It insists that we don't need help, that reaching out is a sign of weakness and a blow to our independence. In the ego's perspective, admitting powerlessness is admitting defeat, which is simply unacceptable.

However, this narrative is deeply flawed and dangerous. Addiction, like any significant challenge in life, is not easily vanquished alone. It's a complex interplay of psychological, physiological, and often socio-environmental factors, which requires comprehensive and often professional intervention to effectively address.

The ego's insistence on maintaining control and refusing help can be likened to a captain refusing to abandon a sinking ship, despite knowing that staying aboard will inevitably lead to disaster. By refusing to admit the reality of the situation, the ego isolates us, cutting us off from the lifelines of support that could pull us from the depths of our struggles.

Moreover, the ego's false narrative of invincibility can lead to a cycle of self-defeat. When we inevitably falter in our solitary fight against addiction, the ego uses these moments as 'proof' of our weakness or failure, driving us deeper into the abyss of self-loathing and despair.

So, how do we break free from this ego-driven narrative?

The key lies in understanding that acknowledging our struggles and reaching out for help is not a sign of weakness but rather an act of strength and courage. It requires immense bravery to be vulnerable, to let others in, and to admit that we need assistance. This act of humility doesn't undermine our power; instead, it enhances it.

Shattering the ego's narrative means recognizing that admitting powerlessness over addiction isn't about giving up; it's about creating space for change. It's about understanding that being human means we are not invincible, and that's perfectly okay. It's about opening ourselves up to the help and support that can guide us along our journey from powerlessness to empowerment.

By challenging the ego's narrative, we allow ourselves to connect authentically with others, to learn from their wisdom and to lean on their support. We transform our journey of recovery from a solitary battle into a shared journey of hope, resilience, and empowerment. This shift is a crucial step toward breaking free from the shackles of addiction and embracing the liberating power of empowerment.

Remember, the ego is not inherently evil. It helps us assert our individuality and aids us in navigating our social world. But in the throes of addiction, it can blind us to our own powerlessness, pushing us further away from the truth and the help we so desperately need. It's a master illusionist, creating a sense of control where there is none. Has your ego ever deceived you in such a way? Have you ever found yourself holding on to control when you should be letting go?

Upon realizing the detrimental role ego plays in one's journey, you must begin to work on taming it by acknowledging powerlessness not as a defeat but as a steppingstone toward recovery. In doing so, you can open yourself up to external help, finally allowing the healing process to commence.

What about you? Are you ready to confront your ego, acknowledge your powerlessness, and open the doors to change? Could surrendering to this fact be the first step toward your recovery?

Remember, acknowledging powerlessness isn't about admitting defeat. It's about admitting that the fight against addiction isn't one you need to wage alone. It's about realizing that you're part of a greater whole, a cosmic web interlinked by mutual support and understanding. It's about realizing that it's okay to ask for help.

How about now? Are you ready to admit your powerlessness over your addiction? Are you ready to surrender your ego, embrace humility, and open yourself up to divine intervention? If so, you are taking the first and most crucial step on the road to recovery.

With the acceptance of powerlessness acting as the key that unlocks the door to a new path, no longer will you be burdened by the weight of ego, and you will discover a newfound sense of freedom. Embracing powerlessness isn't about succumbing to addiction; it is about surrendering the fight to a Higher Power and allowing divine intervention to guide you.

Through surrender, you began to see that you are not alone in your struggle. You become part of a larger community; a collective consciousness bonded by shared experiences. This realization offers a profound sense of connection and unity, replacing the isolation and despair that addiction had once created. Have you ever felt such a profound sense of connection? Have you ever experienced the comfort of shared struggle and the solace it brings?

With this newfound perspective, we can embrace the rest of the Twelve Steps, each one offering further insight and growth. We can move on admitting the exact nature of our wrongs, making amends, seeking guidance through prayer and meditation to improve our conscious contact with God or a Higher Power. Throughout this process, we remain open and humble, our ego no longer a barrier but a bridge to understanding.

Can you envision the power of such a transformation in your life? Can you see yourself breaking down the walls of ego, admitting your wrongs, making amends, and seeking a deeper connection with your spiritual self?

Looking back at my journey, I can't help but acknowledge the role my ego played. It was there in every high and every low, whispering reassurances or doubts that often led me astray. It fed my addictions, promising me control, promising me I was the exception, that I was stronger. My ego led me into relapses, broke my relationships, put me into legal troubles, and even saw me incarcerated, homeless, and left me at death's door with the pleading desperation of a dying man. The suffering was real, and it was immeasurable.

But as I faced these setbacks, each one a blow to my ego, I also saw an opportunity. An opportunity to learn, to reflect, to grow. They made me question my invincibility, my control, my self-centered approach to life. They made me face the reality that my ego had become my own worst enemy.

I had to acknowledge that my ego was the architect of my devastation. It was a difficult pill to swallow. Accepting this was an act of humility, a surrender of my egoistic perspective that had, for so long, blinded me from seeing the truth of my condition. But with each devastating event, my ego began to crumble. The illusion it had so carefully crafted began to fade.

And in its place, I began to clearly see the destructiveness of my addiction, the importance of humility, the value of surrendering. I understood that each setback was not just a failure but a lesson. These setbacks became my greatest teachers, providing invaluable insights into my journey toward recovery.

Every misstep I made, every trouble I encountered, reshaped me. It made me wiser, stronger, more resilient. My ego, once my downfall, became my steppingstone to recovery. I used my past experiences, my struggles, and my sufferings as a tool for understanding myself better and helping others in their journey.

Today, I view my ego differently. It's not my enemy but rather a part of me that needs understanding and taming. It is something I must be always tolerant and aware of. I learned to listen to it, recognize when it's leading me astray, and step back before it sends me spiraling down the same old destructive path.

So, if you are struggling with your ego, remember, it's not about defeating it but about understanding it. It's about learning from the setbacks it might cause and using those lessons to fuel your journey toward recovery.

Could you identify when your ego is taking control? Can you see the valuable lessons hidden within each setback? Can you leverage these experiences to not only further your recovery but also to assist others in theirs? Are you ready to shift your perspective of your ego from an enemy to a guide, a teacher in your recovery journey?

We, as a community in recovery, have a unique opportunity to learn from our struggles and use them as steppingstones on our path to sobriety. Let's shift our perspective on setbacks and see them as opportunities for growth. Let's acknowledge our ego, not as an adversary, but as a part of ourselves that requires understanding and direction.

In this path of recovery, we've discovered that it's not about defeating our ego but rather understanding it, directing it toward a more positive direction. Every setback, every relapse, every struggle gives us a unique insight into our journey and helps us learn more about ourselves. It's not easy, and it's often uncomfortable, but it's a necessary part of our growth.

As we shift our perspective, we begin to see our past failures not as points of shame but as badges of honor—signs that we've learned, grown, and evolved. Our relapses, our legal issues, our relationship troubles become our strength, for they hold the most valuable lessons in our recovery journey.

Moreover, by acknowledging our ego's role in our struggles, we open ourselves up to grace, compassion, and humility—critical components of any recovery journey. The humility to recognize our mistakes, the compassion to forgive ourselves, and the grace to move forward are invaluable gifts that we give ourselves.

So, let's take a moment to reflect: How can you learn from your ego? How can you use your past experiences to not only further your recovery but also to assist others in their journey? Are you ready to embrace the lessons that come with each setback and use them as steppingstones on your path to sobriety?

Remember, this journey of recovery is not a sprint, it's a marathon. It's not about the destination but about the journey. And in this journey, every setback, every struggle, every stumble is a chance for us to grow, learn, and become the best version of ourselves. And isn't that what recovery is all about? Becoming the best version of ourselves despite our struggles, despite our past, despite our ego. We are not defined by our past but by how we choose to move forward. So, let's choose to move forward with grace, compassion, and humility, one step at a time.

The final step in the recovery journey is carrying a message of hope to others who suffer and practicing principles of honesty, love, integrity, unselfishness, and tolerance for others in all our affairs. The final step serves as a message of hope to others who suffer. It is more than a directive; it becomes our life's mission. Can we see how this step, unlike the others, is not about introspection or self-improvement alone? Instead, it is about extending our hand, sharing our journey, our hard-won wisdom and hope with others who are still navigating the stormy waters of addiction.

With each story we share, we find that our past struggles weren't in vain. Each hardship, each setback, had a purpose—it was a lesson that we can now pass on to others. Each scar on our psyche was a signpost, a warning, and a guide for those who follow in our footsteps. Can we comprehend the incredible power of our personal journeys, how every stumble and fall, every victory, has the potential to light the way for others?

When we practice these principles in all our affairs, it isn't merely about maintaining our sobriety. It is about embodying the lessons of humility, honesty, and spirituality that we'd learned throughout our journey. It is about living in a way that constantly reminds us of where we have been, how far we've come, and the responsibility we have to ourselves first and to those who are still on their path. Can we appreciate the ripple effects of our transformation, not only within our lives but in the lives of others, too?

In carrying the message, we find a purpose that is bigger than ourselves. We see that our journey doesn't end with our recovery; instead, it marks a new beginning—a beginning where we can play a role in the recovery of others. Can you see how your journey, marked by your trials and triumphs, can serve as a beacon of hope for others?

In essence, the final step ties all your experiences, lessons, and growth into one purposeful mission. It serves as a constant reminder of your journey and your commitment to serve others. It brings our story full circle, from a struggle with addiction to a message of hope and resilience. Imagine how powerful it is to transform your most significant challenges into your greatest assets. This is something you do not want to miss!

CHAPTER 8

SPIRITUAL LESSONS FROM THE TWELVE STEPS

Looking at the twelve steps from a spiritual perspective allows us to see them as a path toward greater self-understanding, humility, and connection to a power greater than ourselves. Let's break down how each step aligns with different spiritual teachings:

WE ADMITTED WE WERE POWERLESS OVER ALCOHOL—THAT OUR LIVES HAD BECOME UNMANAGEABLE.

The realm of spirituality and the concept of surrender hold great significance. It involves acknowledging our limitations, letting go of our ego-driven desire for control, and embracing a higher power or divine guidance. The first step of admitting powerlessness and recognizing the unmanageability of our lives aligns perfectly with the essence of surrender and acceptance.

CAME TO BELIEVE THAT A POWER GREATER THAN OURSELVES COULD RESTORE US TO SANITY.

This second step corresponds with the belief in a higher power that can help us in our journey of transformation. It's an expression of faith, a key component in many spiritual practices. The second step, "Came to believe that a power greater than ourselves could restore us to sanity," not only encompasses the belief in a higher power but also carries a promise of transformation and restoration. This step is deeply rooted in faith and is considered a crucial component in various spiritual practices.

MADE A DECISION TO TURN OUR WILL AND OUR LIVES OVER TO THE CARE OF GOD AS WE UNDERSTOOD HIM.

This step signifies a total surrender to the divine, an act of faith that is echoed in many spiritual teachings. It also represents the idea of 'letting go and letting God,' a common theme in spirituality. The third step holds profound significance in spiritual practices. It symbolizes a complete surrender to the divine, an act of faith. This step invites us to relinquish our ego-driven will, and trust in a higher power's care and guidance.

MADE A SEARCHING AND FEARLESS MORAL INVENTORY OF OURSELVES.

This step is a profound invitation to embark on a journey of self-discovery and introspection, mirroring the spiritual practice of self-reflection found in many wisdom traditions. It is an act of courage and honesty, as we take a deep and fearless look at ourselves, our actions, and the impact they have had on our lives and the lives of others.

ADMITTED TO GOD, TO OURSELVES, AND TO ANOTHER HUMAN BEING THE EXACT NATURE OF OUR WRONGS.

Step Five reflects the profound spiritual principle of

confession and acknowledgement found in many wisdom traditions. It is a powerful act of purging oneself from guilt and shame, and it is a transformative step toward healing and growth.

WE BECAME WILLING TO LET GOD REMOVE OUR IMPERFECTIONS.

Step Six is about becoming willing and getting ready to humbly ask God or a Higher Power to remove our imperfections. It's a step that carries a lot of weight in the spiritual world. Think about it—pretty much every spiritual teaching out there praises humility, and this step taps into that same idea. In order to ask for some divine intervention to remove our flaws and make us better people, we first have to find humility. We must let go of ego at this step or we will not succeed.

HUMBLY ASKED OUR HIGHER POWER TO REMOVE OUR SHORTCOMINGS.

When we take this step, we're admitting that we're not perfect. We're owning up to our mistakes and acknowledging that we need some help to become the best version of ourselves. By asking for help in this way, we're opening ourselves up to change and growth. We're letting go of the idea that we're in complete control, and we surrender to something greater than ourselves.

MADE A LIST OF ALL PERSONS WE HAD HARMED AND

BECAME WILLING TO MAKE AMENDS TO THEM ALL.

Step Eight involves creating a comprehensive list of all the individuals we have caused harm to and developing a genuine willingness to make amends to each one of them. This significant step harmonizes with essential spiritual principles such as forgiveness, reconciliation, and the act of making things right.

MADE DIRECT AMENDS TO SUCH PEOPLE WHEREVER POSSIBLE, EXCEPT WHEN TO DO SO WOULD INJURE THEM OR OTHERS.

Step Nine takes the process of making amends a step further by actively engaging in direct actions to address the harm we have caused. It involves seeking out the individuals we have harmed whenever feasible, except in cases where doing so would cause further injury to them or others. This step beautifully aligns with the principles of forgiveness, reconciliation, restitution, and personal accountability. This is the step that will set you free.

CONTINUED TO TAKE PERSONAL INVENTORY AND WHEN WE WERE WRONG PROMPTLY ADMITTED IT.

Step Ten involves the ongoing practice of taking personal inventory and promptly admitting our wrongs and encompasses the powerful concepts of constant self-reflection and the humble acknowledgment of our faults. This step brings freedom and separation from our suffering. It is the turning point when we stop fighting our addictions and mental illnesses. Our spiritual awakening and connection have separated us from them.

SOUGHT THROUGH PRAYER AND MEDITATION TO IMPROVE OUR CONSCIOUS CONTACT WITH GOD AS WE UNDERSTOOD HIM, PRAYING ONLY FOR KNOWLEDGE OF HIS WILL FOR US AND THE POWER TO CARRY THAT OUT.

The Eleventh spiritual principle invites us to engage in a personal, reflective dialogue with God or a Higher Power. Notice that the step requires us to pray "only" for knowledge of his will for us and the power or direction to carry out.

HAVING HAD A SPIRITUAL AWAKENING AS THE RESULT OF THESE STEPS, WE TRIED TO CARRY THIS MESSAGE TO ALCOHOLICS AND TO PRACTICE THESE PRINCIPLES IN ALL OUR AFFAIRS.

The Twelfth step marks a turning point in our spiritual journey, shifting focus from personal healing and growth to outward service and support to others. This spiritual awakening is not a singular event but rather an ongoing process of growing self-awareness, humility, compassion, and understanding, fostered through active engagement with the preceding steps. The twelfth step is where the real work in our recovery begins, and it is the work that will lead to a life of freedom if we are willing to do it.

While these steps originated within the context of

Alcoholics Anonymous, their alignment with various spiritual teachings are universal. They provide a roadmap to inner transformation that anyone, regardless of their faith or belief system, can benefit from. Through surrender, self-reflection, honesty, and unselfish service, these steps guide us on a spiritual journey toward healing and self-discovery.

Now, having established the spiritual essence embedded in the twelve steps, it's essential to understand that these principles are not reserved only for those battling addiction or mental illness alone. They are spiritual guidelines that anyone can incorporate into their lives to foster transformation, growth, understanding, and peace.

At the heart of these steps, we find the central theme of surrender. As we explored earlier in, surrender does not mean defeat. Instead, it is a powerful action of letting go of ego and the control we believe we have over life's outcomes. It's about trusting in a higher power, or the universe, or the Dao, or however else you conceptualize a force greater than yourself. This act of surrender can bring immense freedom and peace.

This takes us back to the paradox of powerlessness that we began with. The acceptance of powerlessness leads to empowerment. It is in surrendering to our limitations that we begin to overcome them.

Consider Step One again. It asks us to admit our powerlessness over addiction (or any other problem), suggesting that our lives have become unmanageable. If we were in total control, wouldn't we just stop the behavior causing the unmanageability? But we don't. It's often our very attempts to exert control that exacerbate the problem.

Our ego, the part of us that insists on control and autonomy, resists this acceptance of powerlessness. Yet spiritual teachings and the principles of AA assert that only when we let go of this struggle can we start to experience genuine change.

Ask yourself the following: Where in your life are you holding onto ego and control that could be surrendered? What might happen if you found some humility, admitted powerlessness, and let go? What higher power can you lean into during this process of surrender? Remember, it's not about having all the answers but about being open to the journey, my friends. As you consider these questions, reflect on how the spiritual principles of surrender and acceptance present in the Twelve Steps can bring about transformation in your own life.

Now that we've established the importance of surrender and acceptance, let's delve further into the spiritual aspects of the twelve steps and how they resonate with various spiritual teachings.

Consider Step Two: "Came to believe that a Power greater than ourselves could restore us to sanity." This step doesn't define what this Higher Power is, it leaves room for your personal beliefs and understandings. This could be God, the Spiritual of the Universe, Nature, Buddha, Jesus Christ, Energy, or any entity or force that is larger than our singular existence. It only need make sense to you. This belief in a Higher Power aligns with many spiritual traditions, promoting the idea that we are part of something larger and more profound than our individual selves. How can embracing this belief influence your perspective on your own struggles?

Let's explore Step Two and the possibilities it opens for us. The belief in a Higher Power, in something greater than ourselves, helps to broaden our perspective and gives us a sense of hope and optimism. It suggests that, while we might not have the power within us to overcome our addiction on our own, there is a greater force that can help us regain control and restore our sanity.

In my own journey, I've come to understand that accepting a Higher Power doesn't necessarily mean adopting religious beliefs if those don't resonate with you. For me, God is the collective energy of the universe, the connection between all beings, the invisible thread that binds us together. It is this power, this universal energy, that I turn to for strength, hope, and healing. I strive every day to build a more conscious relationship with him. I pray only for courage, wisdom, and his will or direction for me. I pray for others instead of my own selfish needs. These are the principles that keep me sober and free.

When we accept a Higher Power into our lives, we acknowledge that we don't have all the answers, and that's perfectly okay. We acknowledge that there is a force in the universe that's bigger than our struggles and that we can tap into this force for strength and guidance.

Take a moment to reflect:
What would acknowledging a Higher Power mean for you? How could it change your approach to overcoming your struggles? Can you visualize this force, and does it offer you comfort or a sense of security?

Step Two is a call to humility, to surrender our pride, ego, and admit our need for help. It's also a beacon of hope, a reassurance that we're not alone in our struggle, that there's a force more significant than us that can guide us to sanity. It's the leap of faith that sets the foundation for our recovery journey.

From this perspective, can you see how accepting a Higher Power is not about giving up but about opening ourselves to the possibility of transformation?

Remember, spirituality is a highly personal journey. What's important is that it makes sense to you and it brings you hope, peace, and a sense of interconnectedness that enables you to face your struggles with newfound courage and resilience.

As we continue to explore the spiritual aspects of

the Twelve Steps, keep reflecting on your understanding of a Higher Power and how it can support your recovery journey. It's an ongoing process, a journey of discovery that unfolds as you navigate your path to recovery.

Step Three urges us to make a decision to turn our will and our lives over to the care of God as we understand him. In many spiritual practices, there's a strong emphasis on surrendering our will to the divine, essentially trusting that the universe or Higher Power will guide us toward our best path. It's about releasing the illusion of control and allowing the flow of life to lead us. This is where faith and trust become central. Can you identify an area in your life where surrendering your will could alleviate personal struggle or tension?

Step Three invites us into a deeper level of trust and faith in something greater than ourselves. It takes us a step away from our self-centered behaviors and beliefs and moves us toward a reliance on a Higher Power. This is where we consciously decide to entrust our lives and will into the care of the divine as we perceive it.

You might find that it's one thing to understand this step conceptually but another to genuinely implement it into your life. It's here that we confront our fear of losing control. Our ego often clings to the idea that we can and must control everything about our lives. But this step asks us to question that belief. Is holding onto that control serving us? Or is it a barrier to the serenity and freedom we seek?

Consider for a moment an area in your life where you might be holding on to control too tightly. Is it a relationship that you're trying to manage? An outcome you're trying to control? Can you visualize what might happen if you were to release that grip and allow your Higher Power to guide the way?

Surrender doesn't mean passivity, resignation or failure but an active engagement in life from a different stance. Instead of paddling against the current, we allow the river of life to carry us forward, trusting that our Higher Power knows the path better than we do.

This spiritual principle of surrender can be found in various faith traditions. In Christianity, for instance, it's embodied in the phrase "Not my will, but Thy will be done." In Buddhism, it aligns with the practice of non-attachment. And in Taoism, it's reflected in the concept of wu wei, or effortless action.

Step Three is a powerful testament to the transformative power of surrender. It shifts us from a place of fear and control to a place of trust and acceptance. It's about stepping back and allowing our Higher Power to lead the way, secure in the belief that we are being guided toward our highest good.

So, I ask you again, can you identify an area in your life where surrendering control could bring relief? How might it feel to trust in the wisdom of God or your Higher Power and to allow that trust to guide your actions? Reflect on these questions as you continue your journey through the Twelve Steps and deeper into your spiritual journey.

The Fourth Step, the moral inventory, echoes the principles of reflection and self-awareness that are integral to spiritual growth. For example, Christianity places great importance on faith and self-reflection as pathways to salvation and divine connection. By acknowledging our faults and understanding our patterns, we create an opportunity for change and growth. Reflect on this: what patterns have you noticed in your life that could benefit from self-examination?

Step Four calls for a "searching and fearless moral inventory of ourselves." This soul-searching process encourages us to take an unflinching look at our behaviors, selfishness, dishonesty, fears, attitudes, and motivations. It's about acknowledging our past mistakes, identifying destructive patterns, and understanding how these have contributed to our current circumstances.

Many spiritual traditions underscore the importance of self-awareness and self-examination as crucial steps toward self-improvement and spiritual growth. In Buddhism, meditation is about looking carefully within, which helps you deeply understand how your mind works and how everything keeps changing. In Hindu philosophy, the concept of 'Svadhyaya,' or self-study, is a vital part of the yogic path. The practice of meditation is also common in Christianity, which encourages daily examination and review of the day's events and one's reactions to them to find where God has been present.

With this step, we're not merely wallowing in guilt or regret over past missteps but aiming to learn from them. This process of self-examination helps us recognize recurring patterns that cause us harm and those around us. It is often the case that these patterns keep us stuck in cycles of addictive behavior.

So, consider what patterns in your behavior may be holding you back? Are there recurring situations, reactions, or emotions that seem to fuel your addictive behavior? Recognizing these patterns is the first step toward breaking them. Remember, the aim here is not self-condemnation but self-understanding.

Bringing this awareness into your daily life could be transformative. You might find that with time, you're better able to pause and choose a different course of action when you see these patterns starting to play out. By shedding light on the darkness of our past behaviors, we allow the possibility of change and growth.

The journey of self-discovery might be uncomfortable, even painful at times, but it's a vital part of recovery. It's about facing ourselves honestly, without judgment, fully recognizing our strengths and weaknesses. This isn't easy work, but it's a necessary part of moving forward and a foundational step on the path toward a life of greater serenity and fulfillment.

I invite you to ponder this: How might the practice of self-examination help you better understand yourself? In what ways can identifying your patterns serve as a beacon guiding you toward healthier choices and behaviors? Remember, this is not an exercise in self-criticism, but a step toward self-awareness and, ultimately, self-growth.

As we proceed with Steps Five to Seven, they align with the spiritual practice of confession seen in many religious traditions and the release of guilt or negative energy. By admitting our wrongs, we create space for forgiveness and healing.

Steps Five to Seven involve sharing our moral inventory with another person (Step Five), becoming ready to have our defects of character removed (Step Six), and humbly asking a Higher Power to remove these shortcomings (Step Seven). These steps align closely with many spiritual traditions that emphasize confession, repentance, and transformation.

In Christianity, for instance, the sacrament of confession provides a platform for believers to admit their sins, seek forgiveness, and make a resolution for change. Similarly, in Buddhism, followers practice the confession of downfalls, where they reveal their unskillful actions to the Three Jewels (the Buddha, the Dharma, and the Sangha), expressing remorse and making a commitment to refrain from such actions in the future.

In Step Five, "Admitted to God, to ourselves, and to another human being the exact nature of our wrongs," we're asked to share our moral inventory with another person. This act of vulnerability can be a powerful catalyst for change, promoting self-acceptance, and fostering deeper connections with others. The act of verbalizing our experiences can help us see them in a new light, providing a fresh perspective that can aid in the healing process.

Step Six, "Were entirely ready to have God remove all these defects of character," is about preparing ourselves for change. It involves recognizing and accepting our flaws, but more than that, it's about developing a willingness to let go of these defects, even if they have served as coping mechanisms in the past.

Step Seven, "Humbly asked Him to remove our shortcomings," entails a humble request to our Higher Power to help us overcome our flaws. This step embodies the spiritual principle of humility, and it represents an act of faith and trust in our Higher Power's ability to bring about change in us.

Consider these questions: How does the act of sharing your struggles with another person impact your perspective on your challenges? How ready are you to let go of your old patterns and coping mechanisms? Are you willing to trust a Higher Power to help you change?

These steps are not about self-deprecation or blaming ourselves for our past. Instead, they are about acknowledging our shortcomings, seeking support, expressing willingness for change, and trusting in a power greater than ourselves to help us on our path to recovery. Each step brings us closer to self-improvement and spiritual growth, leading us from the darkness of our past toward the light of a new life of freedom.

Steps Eight and Nine focus on making amends, and they are akin to the spiritual principle of karma - the law of cause and effect. It teaches us that our actions have consequences, and sometimes we need to rectify the negative impacts we've caused.

These steps embrace the concept of making amends, which is central to the teachings of many spiritual and religious traditions and aligns closely with the law of karma. Karma, a concept originating from Indian religions, is the idea that every action we take has consequences that we will eventually have to face. It's a universal law of cause and effect, implying that whatever we put out into the world—whether it's love, hatred, kindness, or cruelty—will eventually return to us.

By accepting responsibility for the harm we've caused others and becoming willing to make amends, we engage with this universal principle. This process isn't just about apologizing; it's about understanding the depth of our actions, experiencing genuine remorse, and, where possible, taking concrete action to right our wrongs.

Making amends has three significant parts. All three of

them are statements and should never include asking for something in return. Here is an example.

State a purpose: "I owe you a direct amends for what I have done."

Take responsibility: "I take full responsibility for the things I have done that has hurt you so deeply."

State your intention: My intention is to right the wrongs I have done with you and mend our relationship.

Making amends can heal relationships. By making amends, we can begin to mend relationships that have been strained or broken due to our past actions. This process can be a significant step toward healing, both for ourselves and those we've hurt. The process of making amends plays a crucial role in our journey to recovery and empowerment. It signifies our genuine desire for change and our willingness to rectify the wrongs our past actions might have caused. It's not just about seeking forgiveness; it's about acknowledging our faults, learning from them, and making a sincere effort to right those wrongs.

Making amends goes beyond merely saying "I'm sorry." It involves understanding the impact of our actions on others, taking responsibility for any hurt or harm caused, and then seeking to repair that damage in whatever way possible. This could be through a heartfelt apology, a commitment to change, or tangible acts to redress the wrongs done.

It's important to note that making amends is not about

seeking absolution or easing our guilt—it's about healing and growth. It's about acknowledging that our past actions, fueled by addiction or mental health struggles, have hurt others, and now, we wish to contribute positively to their lives and our own.

This process, though often challenging, can bring significant healing. For those we've hurt, our sincere efforts to make amends can provide a sense of closure, an opportunity to heal old wounds, and perhaps pave the way for rebuilding trust and mending relationships.

For ourselves, making amends can be a powerful catalyst for personal transformation. It cultivates humility, empathy, and accountability—qualities that strengthen our character and aid in our recovery. It's a poignant reminder that we're not bound by our past mistakes, that we have the capacity for change, for growth, for healing.

However, making amends must be approached with sensitivity and care. We must respect the other person's feelings and readiness to receive our attempts at making amends. It's crucial to prioritize their needs and respect their boundaries. Making amends should never cause further harm or discomfort to those we're seeking to reconcile with.

Also, while making amends is a significant step toward healing, it's important to understand that not everyone will be willing or ready to accept our amends. This can be painful, but it's crucial to remember that we cannot control others' reactions or feelings. What we can control is our sincerity in making amends and our commitment to personal growth and change.

Acknowledging our mistakes and taking responsibility for them is a potent catalyst for personal growth. It is an essential step in our journey toward empowerment, facilitating profound self-awareness, understanding, and, ultimately, transformation.

When we admit our errors, we unmask them. We bring them out of the shadows of denial and into the light of conscious awareness. By doing so, we strip them of their power to control us unconsciously. It's only by facing our mistakes that we can begin to understand them—to learn what led to them, how they impacted us and others, and what they can teach us.

Taking responsibility for our mistakes is a courageous act of self-honesty. It involves acknowledging not only our actions but also their consequences. It's a clear declaration that we are the architects of our actions and that we are ready to own their results, whether they're positive or negative.

By accepting responsibility, we shift from a victim mindset—where we may feel that we are at the mercy of external circumstances or other people's actions—to an empowerment mindset. We recognize that we have control over our decisions, behaviors, and, ultimately, our lives.

This process of acknowledgment and responsibility

allows us to reflect deeply on our actions and their consequences. Reflection provides a mirror, showing us our strengths and weaknesses and highlighting areas for improvement. It encourages introspection, fostering a better understanding of our motivations, fears, desires, and values.

By learning from our mistakes, we turn them into steppingstones rather than stumbling blocks. Each error becomes a lesson, an opportunity for growth and improvement. This learning allows us to make better choices in the future, to evolve, to become more emotionally intelligent and resilient.

Acknowledging our mistakes and taking responsibility for them also nurtures empathy and humility. It helps us recognize and respect the fact that we are all fallible humans who make mistakes. This realization can make us more understanding and compassionate, both toward ourselves and others.

Acknowledging mistakes and taking responsibility fosters trust and authenticity in our relationships. It shows that we are not afraid to be vulnerable, to admit when we're wrong, and to do what it takes to make things right. It builds our character and cultivates respect from others.

In essence, the act of acknowledging our mistakes and taking responsibility for them is a powerful tool for personal growth. It moves us away from blame and excuses and propels us toward understanding, learning, and empowerment. It is a testament to our strength, resilience, and dedication to becoming the best versions of ourselves.

The process of making amends goes beyond personal growth and the healing of individual relationships. It has a wider, more transformative impact that can disrupt and break cycles of harm, fostering healthier dynamics within families, communities, and even society.

The first step in breaking these cycles of harm is acknowledgment. By openly recognizing the harm we've caused, we invalidate the destructive patterns that have perpetuated it. We replace denial and avoidance with conscious awareness, which is crucial for change.

When we make amends, we don't just apologize for our actions; we take active steps to rectify our wrongs. This could involve changing harmful behaviors, rebuilding trust, or even engaging in acts of restitution or reparation. In doing so, we're making a clear commitment to change—a pledge not to repeat our past mistakes. This act itself can interrupt the cycle of harm, replacing it with a cycle of healing and positive change.

Moreover, making amends can prevent further harm by fostering empathy and understanding. As we confront the effects of our actions on others, we become more aware of the impacts of our behavior. This enhanced understanding can deter us from causing similar harm in the future.

Importantly, making amends can also inspire others. As we work to repair the harm we've caused, others may be encouraged to do the same, creating a ripple effect of positive change. It can transform interpersonal dynamics, shift family patterns, and even influence societal norms.

However, it's essential to remember that making amends is a process, not a one-time act. To receive the promise that we stop fighting everything and everyone as found in the Tenth step, we must initially and continually be committed to an ongoing effort. It may involve working through complex emotions, rebuilding broken relationships, and continually striving to be better. It can be challenging, but the rewards—breaking cycles of harm, fostering healing, and promoting personal and collective growth—are immeasurable.

Holding onto guilt and regret can be heavy burdens to bear, often serving as emotional anchors that tether us to our past mistakes. They keep us stuck in a cycle of negative self-judgment, replaying our errors over and over again in our minds and preventing us from moving forward. This cycle can be emotionally exhausting and can hinder our growth and recovery.

Making amends offers us a way to release these burdens. It is an act of self-compassion and forgiveness that allows us to reconcile with our past and create space for healing and peace.

By facing the impact of our past actions and taking steps to rectify them, we replace guilt and regret with responsibility and reparation. This shift helps us to see our past not as a source of shame but as a valuable learning experience. It fosters a sense of closure, affirming that we've done our best to correct our wrongs and that it's now time to move forward.

Making amends also helps us cultivate self-forgiveness, an essential element of inner peace. By acknowledging that we are fallible human beings who make mistakes, but also have the capacity to learn and grow from them, we can extend compassion and forgiveness to ourselves. This does not mean forgetting or excusing our actions but rather accepting them as part of our journey and releasing the self-condemnation associated with them.

When we make amends, we give ourselves permission to let go of the painful emotions tied to our past. We clear the emotional clutter that guilt and regret create, making room for feelings of peace, self-respect, and self-love.

It's important to note, however, that letting go of guilt and regret doesn't happen overnight. It's a process that requires patience, perseverance, and continual self-compassion. There might be moments of relapse, where old feelings of guilt resurface, but these moments do not signal failure. Instead, they are opportunities to reaffirm our commitment to forgiveness and growth.

Making amends is a powerful tool for releasing the burdens of guilt and regret. It enables us to face our past, learn from it, and make positive changes. It encourages self-forgiveness and cultivates inner peace, supporting our journey from a state of emotional turmoil to one of empowerment and serenity.

From a spiritual perspective, making amends aligns with the principle of spirituality. Making amends is an integral aspect of spiritual growth and transformation, aligning with several spiritual principles and teachings. It's an opportunity for redemption, reconciliation, and healing, all of which are central to many spiritual practices. Let's look deeper into the spiritual dimensions of making amends.

PRINCIPLE OF KARMA

As mentioned earlier, the concept of Karma, predominantly found in Eastern philosophies such as Hinduism and Buddhism, implies that every action generates a force of energy that returns to us in kind. When we choose actions that bring happiness and success to others, the fruit of our karma is happiness and success. Therefore, by making amends and rectifying our wrongdoings, we are essentially creating positive karma that can lead to more positive outcomes in our future. It's a process of balancing the scales, of righting the wrongs, to pave the way for a more harmonious future.

PRINCIPLE OF FORGIVENESS

Many spiritual traditions emphasize the importance of forgiveness. In Christianity, for instance, forgiveness is a recurring theme, with teachings encouraging followers to forgive others as God has forgiven them. When we make amends, we seek forgiveness from those we've wronged, but equally important, we also learn to forgive ourselves. Self-forgiveness is a powerful spiritual practice that can lead to profound inner peace and personal growth.

PRINCIPLE OF COMPASSION

Making amends is also deeply connected to the spiritual principle of compassion, a core value in many spiritual traditions, including Buddhism. By making amends, we express empathy and understanding toward those we have hurt, reflecting a compassionate outlook. Simultaneously, it fosters self-compassion as we learn to gently navigate our imperfections and mistakes.

PRINCIPLE OF HUMILITY

Making amends requires humility—acknowledging our faults and the harm we've caused. This humility aligns with various spiritual teachings. In the Islamic tradition, for instance, humility is a highly valued virtue. It allows us to see beyond our ego, accept our fallibility, and understand our place in the grand scheme of things.

PRINCIPLE OF ACCOUNTABILITY AND RESPONSIBILITY

Many spiritual philosophies encourage personal responsibility and accountability for our actions. Making amends embodies this principle. It's about taking ownership of our past mistakes, rectifying them, and committing to avoid repeating them.

PRINCIPLE OF GROWTH AND TRANSFORMATION

Making amends can also be seen as a part of the spiritual journey of personal growth and transformation. Many spiritual paths regard life as a journey of learning and evolution, with mistakes serving as opportunities for growth. By making amends, we not only rectify past errors but also cultivate virtues such as empathy, compassion, humility, and responsibility, facilitating our spiritual evolution.

PRINCIPLE OF HEALING AND RESTORATION

Making amends also resonates with the spiritual principle of healing and restoration. Spirituality often involves the pursuit of wholeness and healing, both within ourselves and in our relationships with others. By making amends, we participate in a powerful process of healing, repairing relationships strained or broken by past actions, and restoring a sense of harmony and unity. It promotes healing not only in the external world but also within our inner self, helping us move past guilt, regret, and self-condemnation.

PRINCIPLE OF LOVE

Love, in its many forms, is a common thread running through numerous spiritual traditions. Making amends is an act of love—love for those we've hurt and also love for ourselves. By taking steps to correct our wrongdoings, we are expressing a deep respect and care for the wellbeing of others, demonstrating an altruistic love. At the same time, allowing ourselves to make mistakes, learn from them, and rectify them is a form of self-love, reflecting a compassionate and understanding relationship with ourselves.

PRINCIPLE OF CONNECTION

Many spiritual philosophies posit that we are all interconnected, part of a larger, intricate web of life. From this perspective, making amends can be seen as a process of restoring broken connections and fostering healthier, more harmonious relationships. It recognizes the ripple effect of our actions, acknowledging that our behaviors impact others and, in turn, the broader web of life.

PRINCIPLE OF ATONEMENT

In some spiritual traditions, such as Judaism, there is a specific principle of atonement, a process of making amends or reparations for harm or wrongs done. Yom Kippur, the Day of Atonement, is a solemn day of repentance and making amends. The act of making amends, in this sense, becomes a deeply spiritual practice tied to penitence, reconciliation, and restoration.

By making amends, we embrace these spiritual principles, inviting positive karma, love, forgiveness, humility, compassion, growth, and transformation into our lives. It's a process of shedding our past burdens, learning from our experiences, and stepping into a future that is not dictated by our past but informed and enriched by it. In essence, making amends is a testament to our capacity for change and our unwavering spirit, reflecting the potential for redemption inherent in all of us. It's a profound act of turning toward the light, a crucial step on our spiritual journey toward a higher, more enlightened state of being.

So, who are the people you've harmed in your life due to your past actions? Are you willing to make amends and take responsibility for the harm you've caused? How might this process of making amends contribute to your personal growth and recovery journey? Remember, this process takes time and requires a great deal of courage, but the freedom and growth it offers are well worth the effort.

The last three steps are about maintaining our spiritual progress by continued self-examination, prayer or meditation (depending on one's beliefs), and service to others. These steps echo many spiritual teachings that promote introspection, connection with the divine, and selfless service as a way to spiritual growth and fulfillment.

Step Eleven says:

"Sought through prayer and meditation to improve our conscious contact with God, as we understood Him, praying only for knowledge of His will for us and the power to carry that out."

This step signifies the maintenance and strengthening of our connection with the Higher Power through prayer or meditation. This step doesn't dictate how you pray or meditate but encourages you to continuously seek to improve your conscious contact with your Higher Power. In various spiritual traditions, prayer and meditation are considered key tools in fostering a deeper connection with the divine. The aim here is not to request specific outcomes but rather to seek the knowledge of the Higher Power's will for us and the strength to carry it out. Can you think of a way in which you can implement this practice in your daily life?

Let's discuss Step Eleven further, which is a call to improve our conscious contact with our Higher Power. It's a beautiful blend of the spiritual practices of prayer and meditation, but it doesn't provide a rigid blueprint to follow. Rather, it invites each of us to connect with our Higher Power in a way that resonates with us. It emphasizes the active pursuit of a deeper, more conscious relationship with that Higher Power, whatever it might be for each of us.

In various spiritual traditions, prayer is often a way of communicating with the divine, expressing gratitude, seeking guidance, or asking for strength. It's a conscious act that allows us to establish a dialogue with the universe, God, or our understanding of a Higher Power. Meditation, on the other hand, is often used as a tool for quietening the mind, seeking inner peace, and cultivating awareness. It can serve as a space where we listen for the divine guidance that our prayers have requested. So how can this step be implemented in daily life?

This might involve setting aside time each day for prayer or meditation. Meditation requires listening. Communication is a two-way street. Consider this; prayer without meditation is like asking for something we really don't want. Daily meditation is essential to full recovery. Some find it beneficial to start their day with this practice, to set a positive tone and intention for the day ahead. Others may find it soothing to end their day with a moment of quiet reflection or prayer. Some might use both, creating bookends of spiritual practice that frame the day.

However, Step Eleven isn't about performing a ritual at specified times only. It's about creating a living, breathing dialogue with your Higher Power, a relationship that evolves and deepens over time. This might mean taking mindful moments throughout the day to connect with your Higher Power, to express gratitude, seek guidance, or ask for strength in the face of challenges. It could also mean trying to bring a greater sense of awareness to everyday tasks and experiences, seeing the divine in the mundane.

Remember, this step encourages improvement, not perfection. It's not about mastering the art of prayer or meditation overnight but about making a commitment to continue deepening this connection with your Higher Power. Step Eleven of the Twelve-Step program invites us to seek a deeper connection with our Higher Power, often defined by individual interpretation. This could be God, the Universe, Nature, or any other concept that symbolizes a power greater than ourselves. The primary tools for forging this connection, as suggested by the step, are prayer and meditation.

Prayer and meditation are akin to the two sides of a conversation with the divine. Prayer is often perceived as the act of talking to the Higher Power, expressing our thoughts, gratitude, desires, and fears. It can serve as a way to articulate our needs and wishes, laying them before the divine with humility and hope.

Meditation, on the other hand, is about quieting our mind, silencing the incessant chatter, and opening ourselves up to receive. It's a form of listening, of being receptive to the guidance, wisdom, or solace that the Higher Power might offer. It enables us to tap into the divine wisdom that lies within and around us, often obscured by the noise of our everyday thoughts.

Incorporating these spiritual practices into our daily routine can enrich our journey of recovery.

Here are some ways you might integrate Step Eleven into your daily life:

DEDICATE SPECIFIC TIMES FOR PRAYER AND MEDITATION

You might find it beneficial to start your day with a moment of prayer, expressing your hopes for the day, asking for guidance, or simply expressing gratitude for another day of life. Ending your day with a meditative practice can also be beneficial, providing a space to reflect, listen, and find peace. These practices can serve as spiritual bookends, grounding your day in spiritual connection.

CREATE MINDFUL MOMENTS THROUGHOUT THE DAY

Step Eleven isn't limited to specific rituals or practices; it's about cultivating an ongoing connection with your Higher Power. This could mean taking a moment of quiet during a busy day to pray or meditate, expressing gratitude for a meal, or seeking guidance during a challenging situation. Try to find moments throughout your day to consciously connect with your Higher Power.

BRING AWARENESS TO THE MUNDANE

The divine isn't confined to lofty realms; it can be found in the ordinary, everyday moments. Try to bring a sense of sacredness to your daily tasks, whether it's doing the dishes, walking the dog, or commuting to work. See these tasks not as chores but as opportunities to connect with the divine, to find joy, and to practice mindfulness.

PRACTICE COMPASSION AND SERVICE

Spirituality is not just about personal growth; it's also about our connections with others. Practicing acts of kindness, compassion, or service can be another way of deepening your relationship with your Higher Power, embodying the divine qualities of love, compassion, and selflessness.

CULTIVATE PRESENCE

A crucial part of improving our conscious contact with our Higher Power lies in cultivating presence. Often, our minds are occupied with thoughts of the past or worries about the future, disconnecting us from the present moment, which is the only moment where life truly unfolds. By practicing mindfulness, we become more present and open to the divine guidance that often gets drowned out by our mental chatter.

CULTIVATE AN ATTITUDE OF GRATITUDE

An attitude of gratitude can be a powerful tool for enhancing our connection with our Higher Power. Taking a few moments each day to acknowledge and express gratitude for the blessings in our lives—no matter how big or small—can foster a sense of abundance and joy. This practice aligns us with the positive aspects of our existence, opening us up to the goodness of the universe.

ENGAGE IN SPIRITUAL STUDY

Engaging with spiritual texts, philosophies, or teachings can provide insights and guidance to deepen our understanding of the divine. Spiritual study can take many forms, from reading sacred texts to attending spiritual talks or workshops, participating in study groups, or even listening to spiritual podcasts. It invites us to explore different perspectives and continually learn and grow on our spiritual journey.

NURTURE YOUR INNER SANCTUARY

Creating a dedicated space at home for prayer and meditation can help support your spiritual practice. This could be a quiet corner of a room, a small altar, or an entire room if space allows. Fill this space with items that inspire serenity and spiritual connection, such as candles, incense, spiritual symbols, or images. This designated space can serve as your inner sanctuary, inviting you into a state of peace and reverence each time you enter.

NATURE AS A GATEWAY

Nature holds a profound capacity to connect us with the divine. Spending time in nature—be it a walk in a park, a hike in the forest, or simply sitting by a body of water—can facilitate a deeper sense of connection with our Higher Power. The tranquility, beauty, and intricacy of nature can inspire awe and reverence, fostering a sense of oneness with the divine.

Step Eleven invites us into an ongoing journey, a continuous process of deepening our relationship with our Higher Power. It is not a destination but a path, a spiritual practice that evolves and grows over time. And remember, there is no right or wrong way to engage with this step. It's about finding what resonates with you, what nourishes your soul, and what supports you on your journey from powerlessness to empowerment. Every step forward, no matter how small, is a testament to your courage, commitment, and strength. Each day, each moment presents a new opportunity to connect with your Higher Power, to seek guidance, express gratitude, and listen for the divine whispers that guide you on your path.

Finally, Step Twelve states: "Having had a spiritual awakening as the result of these steps, we tried to carry this message to alcoholics, and to practice these principles in all our affairs."

In essence, this step is about service and compassion—foundational virtues in many spiritual paths. It's the embodiment of the spiritual principle that we rise by lifting others. Having experienced the transformative power of the Twelve Steps, we are then asked to act as a beacon for others who are struggling.

This final step points to a common thread woven through many spiritual traditions—the transformation from a self-centered to a service-oriented life. This aligns with the wisdom traditions that teach us that we find meaning, purpose, and deep satisfaction in life not through relentless self-seeking but through self-giving.

Through this lens, the Twelve Steps can be seen as not only a roadmap out of addiction but also a spiritual journey, guiding us toward a life of surrender, self-examination, and service. The process invites us to acknowledge our limitations, to trust in a power greater than ourselves, to embark on a journey of self-discovery and make amends where needed, and finally, to be of service to others.

By seeing the twelve steps from this spiritual lens, we can see how they provide a framework not only for overcoming addiction but also for fostering a deep, lasting change that promotes a holistic, spiritual way of living.

As we've seen, these principles align with many spiritual teachings, encouraging us to surrender, accept, and grow. How might these spiritual insights reshape your understanding of your own journey? Step Twelve represents the culmination of the transformative journey of the Twelve-Step program. Having undergone the spiritual awakening resulting from the preceding steps, we are called to extend our newfound wisdom and strength to others grappling with addiction. This step places a strong emphasis on service and compassion—cornerstones of many spiritual traditions—illuminating a critical shift from self-centeredness to a service-oriented life.

The practice of service, central to Step Twelve, is deeply rooted in spiritual wisdom. Many spiritual traditions affirm that the purpose of life is not merely self-aggrandizement but self-transcendence. It's about shifting our focus from 'me' to 'we,' recognizing that our well-being is intrinsically connected to the well-being of others.

As we offer our support and share our experience, strength, and hope with others struggling with addiction, we not only aid them in their journey but also reinforce our own sobriety and spiritual growth. In this mutual exchange, we see firsthand the spiritual principle: we rise by lifting others. As we assist others, we also help ourselves.

This active practice of service can take many forms, from sponsorship within the Twelve-Step program to simply lending an empathetic ear to those in need. It's about making ourselves available to others, reminding them that they are not alone, and providing hope through our own lived experiences.

Moreover, Step Twelve urges us to practice these principles in all our affairs. This calls for a holistic integration of the lessons learned into every aspect of our lives. The journey of recovery doesn't stop at overcoming addiction; it extends into how we relate to ourselves, others, and the world around us.

This practice leads to a spiritual and psychological transformation that is vital for long-term sobriety. Sobriety is not just about abstaining from substance use—it's about leading a fulfilling, meaningful life. As we embody the principles of the Twelve Steps, we create a life that is rich in purpose, connection, and spiritual depth, a life that supports our continued sobriety.

The importance of Step Twelve in maintaining long-term sobriety cannot be overstated. It serves as a powerful reminder of our journey, keeping the memory of our struggles fresh while highlighting the transformative power of the Twelve Steps. It fosters resilience, humility, and empathy, equipping us with the psychological and spiritual tools necessary to navigate life's challenges without resorting to substance use.

The Twelfth Step will guide us from a state of powerlessness and confusion to a place of empowerment and clarity. It invites us to surrender, to self-examine, to make amends, and ultimately, to serve others, providing a pathway toward a life of meaning, serenity, and fulfillment. As we journey through the steps, we cultivate a spiritual lifestyle that supports long-term sobriety, personal growth, and the deep, lasting change necessary for a fulfilling life.

CHAPTER 9

THE JOURNEY FROM POWERLESSNESS TO EMPOWERMENT

The journey from a state of powerlessness to empowerment is not a linear one, and it often involves stumbling, falling, and rising again. It's a journey that requires perseverance, patience, resilience, and an unflinching belief in one's potential for transformation. The journey starts by recognizing our weaknesses, our struggles, and the truth about our addictions and mental illnesses.

Let's delve deeper into this transformative path. The first step in any journey of transformation is acknowledgment. In the context of addiction and mental health, it means recognizing and admitting that we are powerless over the behavioral and physical aspects of our addictions or mental health issues. This step is far from disempowering; in fact, it can be an act of liberation. If we have a profound Step One experience, it will free us from the false notion that we must be always in control. This acknowledgment isn't a surrender to our condition; instead, it's a surrender to reality—a crucial first step in breaking the cycle.

Once we acknowledge our powerlessness, the second step is to understand that it's okay to seek help. There's great strength in reaching out to a higher power and to others, be they professionals, support groups, or trusted loved ones. This support offers guidance, wisdom, and the practical tools needed for overcoming addiction or managing mental health challenges.

With the support of a Higher Power and from others, we can start rebuilding our belief in ourselves. This involves changing our internal narrative, replacing self-defeating thoughts with empowering beliefs. It involves visualizing our lives free from the chains of addiction or the weight of mental illness. It's about fostering hope, resilience, and the unwavering belief in a power greater than ourselves to give us the strength to change our lives.

Empowerment is not just a feeling; it's a call to action. It involves making difficult but necessary changes in our lives. This might include adopting healthier habits, setting boundaries, practicing mindfulness, daily prayer and meditation, and helping others who suffer. Each small action, when taken consistently, leads us further down the path to empowerment.

We need to take the time to celebrate our victories. Even small victories on our journey should be celebrated. Every step forward, no matter how small, is a sign of progress. Celebrating these victories can help build momentum and reinforce the belief in our ability to change.

Empowerment comes from realizing that our struggles and victories are not just about us. They can serve as beacons of hope for others on similar journeys. By sharing our stories and offering support to others, we not only strengthen our own resolve but also spread empowerment to those still battling their demons.

The path from powerlessness to empowerment is not an easy one, but it is deeply rewarding. It's a journey that calls on us to be honest, brave, compassionate, and resilient. But most importantly, it's a journey that teaches us the incredible strength we hold within us—a strength that not only empowers us but also has the power to inspire and empower others. As we rise from the ashes of our struggles, we become symbols of hope, resilience, and the transformative example of empowerment.

In the Dao De Jing, there's a beautiful expression of this concept: "To yield is to be preserved whole. To be bent is to become straight. To be empty is to be full." The idea is that acknowledging our weaknesses and limitations is not a form of surrender but rather an opening to greater strength. Our vulnerability becomes our strength, our powerlessness an avenue to empowerment.

We need to be mindful of another concept called the Law of Attraction. The main principal of the Law of Attraction is that our thoughts and feelings shape our reality. If we shift our energy from negative to positive, we can attract more positive experiences into our lives. This shift begins with acknowledging our current state. When we accept our powerlessness, we make room for positive energy to enter and shape our journey to recovery.

The journey from powerlessness to empowerment, therefore, is not a linear process. It requires continuous self-examination, surrender, acceptance, and growth. It's about realizing that even though we cannot control everything, we have immense power over how we respond to our circumstances.

As we progress through our journey to recovery, we gradually replace our sense of powerlessness with a growing sense of personal and spiritual empowerment. By seeking help, making amends, continuously self-evaluating, praying, meditating, and helping others, we align ourselves with higher values and a larger purpose, transforming our lives in the process.

In essence, the path from powerlessness to empowerment is a spiritual journey. It's a transformative process that requires us to let go of our egos, embrace humility, and open ourselves up to the guidance of a Higher Power. It invites us to believe in ourselves, to understand that we have the capacity to change, to grow, and to become better versions of ourselves.

The journey is challenging, but the rewards are immeasurable. Can you imagine your journey from powerlessness to empowerment? What does it look like, and what steps are you willing to take to embark on this journey?

We let go of our anxieties and fears and hand them over to a Higher Power, believing in its ability to guide us in the right direction. This isn't about passive resignation or forfeiting control over our lives. Instead, it is about collaborating with the divine, merging our personal will with the spiritual will. Our journey becomes less about fighting our weaknesses and more about celebrating our strengths, less about fear and more about faith.

Take a moment and reflect: How can you align your personal will with your Higher Power? What changes can you make today to practice this act of surrender?

The twelfth step, which involves carrying the message to other alcoholics and practicing these principles in all our affairs, embodies the principles of service, humility, and gratitude. Service to others is a common thread in many spiritual teachings. Whether it's Karma Yoga in Hinduism or the Christian concept of 'agape' (selfless love), serving others is often considered a path to spiritual evolution.

By reaching out to others who are also struggling, we're not just providing them with support but are also fortifying our spiritual foundation. The act of helping others navigate their path reinforces our understanding of the principles of AA and strengthens our resolve. By giving, we receive. By teaching, we learn.

Ask yourself a question: How can I embody the principle of service in my recovery journey? How can my experience be a beacon of hope for others?

When we look at our journey through these lenses, we realize that admitting powerlessness is not the end but the beginning of a transformative journey. It's a path that takes us from a place of darkness and despair to a realm of hope, healing, and spiritual enlightenment. A journey from powerlessness to profound empowerment.

When we truly embrace these teachings and integrate them into our lives, we begin to see the changes they bring. They guide us from a state of powerlessness over alcohol to a state of empowerment, allowing us to break the chains of addiction and reclaim control over our lives. Remember, this journey is not a sprint but a marathon. It requires patience, courage, and a great deal of humility.

Embracing the journey from powerlessness to empowerment also requires us to transform our outlook on life and our relationships with others. It's about moving from isolation to connection, from self-centeredness to selflessness. We start by acknowledging our own frailties, and then we extend that understanding to others, fostering empathy and compassion in our interactions. In the process, we also learn to forgive, both ourselves and others.

Ask yourself, "How has my perspective on life and relationships changed since I started this journey? Have I been able to cultivate more empathy and compassion?"

Similarly, our relationship with ourselves undergoes a significant transformation. Instead of harsh self-criticism and guilt, we start embracing self-love and self-acceptance.

We understand that our mistakes and shortcomings do not define us. They are just parts of our journey, steppingstones toward our growth.

Pause and reflect: How has your self-perception changed since you acknowledged your powerlessness over addiction? Can you find space for self-love and self-acceptance in your heart?

Finally, it's crucial to remember that this journey from powerlessness to empowerment is unique for each person. The pace, the experiences, the challenges—they're different for everyone. So, there's no need to compare your journey with others'. You are on your own path to a full recovery.

At the brink of despair, I experienced the desperation of a dying man. I felt myself sinking deeper and deeper into the dark abyss of addiction and severe mental illness. My life was a never-ending cycle of delusional thinking, daily physical cravings, and withdrawals, punctuated by short-lived highs that left me feeling even more hollow. I had spent so much time chasing sobriety, attending meetings, with short lengths of sobriety, and yet here again, I found myself at death's door. In my desperation, I clung on to the last straw of hope—the remembrance of Step One, admitting my powerlessness and unmanageability of my life.

In this desolate state of the desperation of a dying man, I finally understood my powerlessness. I began to grasp the stark reality—my life, as I had known it, was slipping away. My children were to be left alone without a father. I had nothing left to give or grasp ahold of. But within this darkness, I also found a glimmer of hope. The path out of this despair was not through denying my condition or through willpower alone but through admitting my powerlessness and surrendering to God. It was this place that led me to the fully conceding moment of a spiritual surrender. You see, up to this point in my life, I never fully understood that I couldn't surrender to a higher power until I experienced a profound acceptance that I had the disease of addiction and mental illness first.

Just as the Dao De Jing says, "To hold on to the submissive is called being strong." I embraced this philosophy, understanding that my strength didn't lie in fighting my addiction head-on but in acknowledging my powerlessness, surrendering my control, and opening myself to the healing power of God.

By acknowledging my powerlessness, I shifted my energy from resistance to acceptance, creating space for positive energy to flow into my life. This shift in perspective allowed me to manifest a more positive path.

There's an incredible amount of power that comes from understanding and accepting our own limitations. For me, a realization of the Law of Attraction reinforced my understanding and opened up a whole new world of possibilities.

I had been locked in a battle with my addiction and mental illness, constantly resisting, fighting, and exhausting myself in the process all the way to my death. I was solely focused on what I didn't want—my addiction—and as I had learned; what we focus on tends to be what we attract into our lives. My energy was entirely consumed by my struggle with my addition and mental illness, leaving little room for anything positive to enter.

The moment I truly accepted my powerlessness over my addiction and mental illness, I experienced a profound shift in my energy. It was as if a huge burden had been lifted from me. I no longer had to fight or resist because I had acknowledged and accepted my reality. This was not a sign of defeat but rather a moment of immense courage and strength.

Acceptance, as I learned, creates a mental and emotional space for change. Once I accepted my powerlessness, I was able to shift my focus and energy toward recovery. We attract what we focus on, and for the first time, I was focusing on positive change, on healing, on sobriety.

The Law of Attraction states that like attracts like. By focusing on my desire to heal and to live a life of sobriety, I began to attract positive energy and opportunities that supported my recovery. New doors opened for me. I found myself surrounded by people who encouraged and supported my journey. I began to experience moments of peace and clarity that had been absent during my struggle with addiction.

Through acceptance of my powerlessness, I found empowerment. The shift in my energy and focus allowed the universe to support me on my path to recovery. It wasn't a magic solution to all my problems, but it set me on a journey of healing and growth.

Each step forward on this path felt like a journey from darkness to light, from hopelessness to hope. Each day of sobriety felt like a victory, a testament to my strength and resilience. Each personal connection I made along the way, each helping hand I reached out for, each helping hand I extended, made me feel more grounded, more human.

Over time, I could feel myself transforming. I was no longer a dying man clinging to desperation but a man reborn with a new sense of purpose and direction. My powerlessness over alcohol had led me to a spiritual awakening and personal empowerment that I had never experienced before.

This journey, however, was not an overnight transformation. It required persistence, patience, and commitment. It required me to work through the Twelve Steps of AA, to learn and internalize the teachings of the Dao De Jing and The Secret, teachings by great authors and spiritual leaders, mentors who had been where I was. Most importantly, I had to keep faith and pray for courage to see it through even when the path seemed daunting.

The journey from powerlessness to empowerment is

a path of continual growth and transformation. But the rewards—a life of freedom from addiction or mental illness, a life of purpose and connection, a life worth living—make every step worth it.

Embracing powerlessness, admitting to ourselves that we have no control over our addictions and mental illness, is not an act of defeat but rather the first crucial step toward reclaiming our lives. It marks the beginning of a transformative journey that requires courage, humility, and above all, an unwavering faith in our ability to change and a Higher Power's ability to aid us in that change.

With each step forward, we realize that what began as an admission of powerlessness over our addiction has morphed into an empowering journey of self-discovery and spiritual growth. This transformation doesn't just free us from the chains of addiction; it gifts us a new perspective, a new way of living, that is filled with purpose, gratitude, and serenity.

Yet, this journey, as fulfilling as it may be, is not a destination. It is an ongoing process that continues long after we've taken our last drink. For recovery isn't about 'curing' our addiction but about continuously growing, learning, and finding new ways to live a fulfilling, sober life.

So, I ask you. Are you prepared to keep journeying, keep exploring, keep evolving, even when the path becomes challenging? Are you ready to transform your powerlessness into an empowering journey of spiritual growth and recovery? Will you, like the phoenix, rise from the ashes of your addiction and soar toward a life of freedom and fulfilment?

As we navigate this journey from powerlessness to empowerment, we do so with the understanding that addiction, like life, is not a static state. It ebbs and flows, presenting new challenges and opportunities for growth at every turn. Each step we take is an affirmation of our commitment to ourselves and our recovery. And each day we stay sober is a testament to the incredible inner strength we possess, strength we might have never discovered had it not been for our struggles with addiction.

In this journey, our greatest ally is the acceptance of our powerlessness over alcohol or our addiction. In acknowledging our limitations, we begin to dismantle the destructive forces of denial and resistance that have perpetuated our addictive behaviors. Like a seed buried in the earth, we must surrender to the darkness of our circumstances before we can begin to grow toward the light.

At this point, I'd like you to reflect on your own journey so far. How have you transformed since admitting your powerlessness? How has surrendering control led to moments of growth in your life? In what ways have you experienced empowerment through your recovery process?

As we walk this path, we discover that the principles

found in the twelve steps are not isolated strategies meant solely for dealing with addiction. They are, in fact, profound spiritual tenets that can guide us in all aspects of life. They remind us of the importance of honesty, humility, restitution, mindfulness, prayer, and service—values that are deeply rooted in almost every spiritual tradition.

And just like the Law of Attraction, the Twelve-Step program also echoes the same fundamental truth; the energy we radiate, the thoughts and beliefs we hold about ourselves and the world, have a powerful influence on our reality. As we change our thinking, we begin to change our lives.

In essence, the journey from powerlessness to empowerment is not just about overcoming addiction but a journey of spiritual awakening and personal transformation. It is about discovering our true selves, understanding our place in the universe, and recognizing our inherent worth. It is about moving away from the shackles of our past and stepping into a life filled with hope, love, and endless possibilities.

So, let's continue this journey together, supporting one another, learning from each other, and celebrating each step we take toward empowerment and recovery. Remember, you are not alone in this journey. We are all in this together. The question is, are you ready to take the next step?

Taking this journey of recovery is much like embarking

on a long, adventurous trek. It is not merely about reaching the destination; it is about every step taken, every hardship overcome, every moment of joy experienced, and every lesson learned along the way. In recovery, like in a trek, the terrain will vary; it can be smooth and peaceful at times and rough and tumultuous at others. What's important, however, is that we keep moving forward, no matter how slow the progress may seem.

One of the most vital aspects of this journey is patience. Healing takes time. Personal growth takes time. Spiritual awakening takes time. A journey of a thousand miles begins with a single step. It is essential for us to remember that our recovery journey is not a race; there is no finish line to cross. It is an ongoing process of self-discovery and healing.

Next, I would like to bring your attention to a crucial part of our journey—the inevitable setbacks and challenges we will face. There will be days when we stumble, days when we fall back into old patterns. These moments are not failures. They are opportunities for learning, for growth, for gaining a deeper understanding of ourselves and our triggers. Remember, even in moments of relapse, we are not starting over; we are starting from experience. How do you perceive setbacks in your recovery? How can you use them as steppingstones toward personal and spiritual growth?

Lastly, let's not forget the power of community on this journey. The fellowship in AA, the shared experiences, the unconditional support, and love—these are pillars upon which we can lean when the journey gets hard. There is immeasurable strength in knowing that we are not alone, that there are others who understand our struggles, our fears, and our hopes.

The journey from powerlessness to empowerment is a deeply transformative, profoundly spiritual, and uniquely personal journey. It is about embracing our vulnerabilities, about transforming our struggles into strengths, and about evolving from a state of despair and hopelessness to a life filled with hope, peace, and sobriety. Remember, every step taken on this journey, no matter how small, is a step toward a better, healthier, and more fulfilling life. How are you feeling about this journey? Are you ready to embrace the challenges and triumphs that lie ahead?

CHAPTER 10

EMBRACING THE POWER OF NOW

The acknowledgment of our own powerlessness may at first seem like an admission of defeat. But in truth, it is a bold declaration of honesty, a fundamental cornerstone of personal growth and spiritual awakening. This journey that we've explored illuminates a profound truth: that true power is often found in places where we least expect it—in surrender, in acceptance, in the present moment.

One of the greatest hurdles we face in our journey toward empowerment and recovery is the formidable barrier of the ego. The ego clings to self-will, stubbornly insisting on maintaining control even when this control is clearly causing harm and leading us astray. It resists admitting powerlessness, viewing such an admission as a threat to its very existence.

But what happens when we release this ego-driven need for control? What happens when we embrace our limitations, not with resentment but with acceptance and even gratitude?

Embracing our limitations in the present moment is like finding the key to a prison cell in which we've long been confined. It frees us from the self-imposed shackles of ego and self-will, allowing us to step into a more conscious, enlightened existence.

When we release our rigid attachment to self-will and instead lean into the wisdom of a Higher Power, we open ourselves up to guidance that can lead us down a path of true empowerment. It is in this act of surrender that we find freedom—not a freedom to do whatever we want but a freedom to do what is best for our growth, healing, and ultimate wellbeing.

In *The Power of Now,* spiritual teacher Eckhart Tolle speaks about the liberation that comes from living fully in the present moment, detached from past regrets and future anxieties. This is the space where true change happens. It's in the now that we can fully experience and accept our reality, learning from our past without being enslaved by it and planning for our future without being consumed by it.

Consider this: in what ways might your life change if you fully embraced the power of now? If you surrendered your self-will and acknowledged your limitations, not as barriers but as steppingstones on the path to a more conscious, enlightened existence? This isn't an easy path to tread, but the rewards are profound. Embracing our powerlessness in the present moment can truly set us free, providing a solid foundation for a journey of continuous growth and spiritual awakening.

As we continue down this path of acceptance and surrender, we begin to experience a shift. The perceived weakness of admitting powerlessness transforms into a source of strength. Our limitations, once seen as obstacles, are now regarded as opportunities for growth. Our perspective alters and we realize the value of the present moment—the only place where true change can occur.

Can you feel the shift happening within you? Can you sense how your perspective of powerlessness is changing? Perhaps you are beginning to understand the strength inherent in surrender and the liberation that it brings.

We also begin to comprehend how much energy we were expending in futile attempts to control the uncontrollable. We understand how this struggle was depleting us, preventing us from fully living in the 'now.' By ceasing this struggle, we recover this energy. We can then channel it into living fully in the present, connecting with our Higher Power, and making positive changes in our lives.

This transition isn't a linear path; it's more akin to a winding road with its fair share of ups and downs. There might be moments of doubt, moments when the ego tries to regain control. And that's okay. It's part of the process. Can you forgive yourself for these moments and see them as opportunities for learning and growth, rather than as setbacks?

Embracing the 'Power of Now' means accepting everything that the present moment contains—the good and the bad, the easy and the difficult. It's about being fully present with whatever arises without judgment or resistance. This acceptance allows us to learn, grow, and evolve.

The path of recovery, of moving from powerlessness to empowerment, is not easy. It takes courage, faith, and a great deal of honesty. Yet, it is a journey that promises profound transformation. By acknowledging our powerlessness and surrendering to a Higher Power, we pave the way for a life of peace, fulfillment, and true empowerment.

In this journey, it is essential to remember that you are not alone. As you navigate through the valleys and peaks, remember that there is a community around you, ready to hold your hand and walk this path with you. They too have wrestled with the tumultuous seas of powerlessness and emerged stronger, more aware, and truly empowered. Are you willing to lean into this support and learn from the shared experiences of others?

It's also crucial to note that this path is not a destination but an ongoing process of growth and discovery. Each day, each moment, offers a new opportunity to choose surrender over control, acceptance over resistance, love over resentment, and faith over fear. Can you see the power in each moment of your journey? Can you embrace the potential for transformation that exists in every instant?

Embracing our powerlessness and living in the 'now' also enables us to tap into a deep well of inner strength that we may not have known existed. It allows us to align with our Higher Power, enabling us to move through life's challenges with grace, courage, and resilience. As we cultivate this connection with our Higher Power, we find an endless source of support, guidance, and wisdom.

Indeed, the journey from powerlessness to empowerment is not a linear path but more akin to a spiral. At times, it may feel as if you're going in circles, wrestling with the same challenges, the same feelings of powerlessness. But remember, each time you confront these challenges, you do so with increased wisdom, deeper insight, and a stronger connection to your Higher Power. You're not moving in circles but spiraling upward, each loop taking you closer to the person you aspire to be.

Remember, your path is unique. It's not meant to be compared to anyone else's. It's not a race. It's about finding your rhythm, your pace, and trusting that you are exactly where you need to be.

Accept your journey as it is, without judgement or comparison.

In the Dao De Jing, it says, "The journey of a thousand miles begins with one step." You have taken many steps on your journey, some small, some giant leaps. Each step, no matter its size, is a victory. Each step is an act of courage, an affirmation of your commitment to growth and transformation.

So, as we move forward, let us celebrate each step, each moment of surrender, each instance of acceptance.

Let's recognize them for what they truly are—powerful acts of faith and humility, integral to our journey toward empowerment.

Embrace each step of your journey with gratitude, recognize your growth, and celebrate your victories, no matter how small. Continue this journey, with all its twists and turns, trusting in your Higher Power and the wisdom of the process.

The path from powerlessness to empowerment is not an easy one, but the rewards are immeasurable. You're not only reclaiming your life but transforming it into something more meaningful, fulfilling, and beautiful than you ever imagined.

Remember, you are not alone. You have your Higher Power, your community, and your own indomitable spirit guiding you along the way. With each step you take, you are growing stronger, more empowered, more aligned with your true self. So, keep going, keep growing, and keep embracing the power of now.

As we wrap up, let's reflect once more on how far you've come and how far you can go. Acknowledging our powerlessness is not about accepting defeat or succumbing to our struggles. Rather, it's about accepting the reality of our situation and recognizing that we need help.

Think back on your own journey, the times when you felt powerless. Now, think about how those moments have shaped you, led you to seek help, to make changes.

They were not moments of weakness but turning points, leading you toward strength and growth. Can you now see the strength in your vulnerability? The courage in your surrender?

Embracing the power of now, as Eckhart Tolle teaches us, involves fully accepting this moment as it is, without wishing it were different. When we stop resisting what is, we create space for transformation to occur. Consider this: How has living in the present moment shifted your experience of powerlessness? How has it shaped your journey toward empowerment?

By being fully present, we disengage from our past mistakes and future worries, we anchor ourselves in the present, the only place where life truly happens. The present moment is where we find our power, where we make choices that shape our lives. Can you recall a moment when you chose to be fully present? How did that impact your journey of recovery and self-discovery?

Your journey from powerlessness to empowerment is not just about overcoming addiction or other challenges. It's a spiritual journey, a journey of personal growth and transformation. It's about becoming the best version of yourself, about living a life of purpose and fulfillment.

As we close, I'd like you to remember that your journey is not over. It's a continuous process of growth and transformation. But with each step you take, with each moment of surrender, you are moving closer to your true self, to a life of empowerment, fulfillment, and peace.

Continuing with your journey of transformation and growth, the next step is one of continual awareness and diligence. Even as you progress, there will be moments of doubt, moments of weakness, and moments of temptation. This is all part of the journey. It's not a linear path, but rather a cycle of growth and learning. What are some challenges you foresee in your future? How can the principles of powerlessness, surrender, and living in the present moment assist you in those times? And, importantly, how will you celebrate your victories, both big and small, along the way?

Embracing the power of now is about acknowledging that all you truly have is this moment. It's about giving up the illusion of control over the past and the future and instead focusing your energy on what you can control—your actions and attitude right now. This realization is freeing and empowering. You are not bound by your past mistakes or future worries. You have the power to shape your life, one moment at a time.

How will you use this moment, right now, to continue your journey of growth and transformation? What is one small step you can take today that will move you closer to your goals? How will you incorporate the principles of powerlessness and surrender into your daily life?

The teachings and promises found within the Twelve Steps and from other authors are just guides along your path. Ultimately, the journey is yours. You hold the power to change, to grow, to overcome your struggles. You hold the power to shape your life and become the person you want to be.

Keep going, keep learning, keep growing. You are not powerless over your life. In fact, you are incredibly powerful. By surrendering to the flow of life and embracing the power of now, you are opening yourself up to endless possibilities.

As we conclude our journey today, I invite you to reflect on your experiences and insights. Consider the steps you've taken and the progress you've made. And as you move forward, I encourage you to continue practicing these principles in all aspects of your life, embracing the power of the present moment, and living in conscious contact with your Higher Power.

Are you ready to take the next step in your journey toward empowerment? Will you continue to surrender, to accept, to grow? Will you choose a life of conscious connection, present awareness, and true freedom? The choice, my friends, is yours.

I hope this book has been enlightening for you. My hope and prayers are that each and every one of you who suffer from life issues, addiction or mental health issues will find peace and serenity.

As I bid farewell today, I yearn to impart the precious words of wisdom bestowed upon me by my father during his time on this earth. If you spend your life selfishly pursuing worldly possessions, never sharing, never giving to others, your good name shall fade into oblivion, lost and forgotten. But if you choose to live your life with honesty, integrity, compassion, and love for your fellow beings, you shall weave a legacy that transcends the bounds of time.

In the days that lie ahead, I hope for a destined reunion, whether in this realm or the hereafter, where I can clasp your hand and utter, "Well done, my friend, well done!"

Robert Beatty

CHAPTER 11

STORIES OF REDEMPTION

EMILY'S STORY

I never thought my life could be redeemed from the depths of despair. As a child, I suffered unthinkable abuse that scarred my soul. The pain was like a wildfire consuming everything in its path, leaving behind only ashes and brokenness. The darkness that enveloped my young heart led me down a treacherous path of addiction. But through a divine connection with God, I discovered the strength to rise above my demons and forge a new path of redemption—a path that would ultimately lead me to help others who were still trapped in the clutches of addiction.

My earliest memories are tainted by fear and violence. I grew up in a home where love was a foreign concept and safety was an unattainable dream. My father, a slave to his own addictions, unleashed his anger on our family with a brutality that knew no bounds. I became a receptacle for his pain, an outlet for his rage. With each passing day, the wounds deepened, and my innocence was stolen away.

The only respite I found from the harsh realities of my existence was in the arms of addiction. It offered me temporary solace, an escape from the haunting memories that plagued my every waking moment. Drugs became my sanctuary—a twisted refuge that momentarily numbed the pain but left me more broken than before.

For years, I spiraled down a path of self-destruction. My life became a chaotic dance between the pursuit of the next high and the depths of despair that inevitably followed. Friends and family watched helplessly as I slipped further into the abyss, my spirit fading away like a dying ember until I found myself homeless, addicted to heroin, and prostituting myself as a means to feed my addiction and sustain the meager existence of my reality.

But even in the darkest of nights, a flicker of hope always remained. Something I fundamentally knew and refused to reach for. It was during my lowest moment that I found myself brutally beaten, hospitalized in intensive care, hanging on to what life I had left, that I finally felt a profound connection with something greater than myself. In this state, I had nothing more to give in my life other than a simple prayer. The words uttered under my shaking voice.

"Take me, please..."

It was as if a divine hand reached down and cradled me in my despair. In that moment, I discovered God—a presence that saw past my brokenness and loved me unconditionally. For the first time in my life, I knew everything was going to be okay.

With newfound faith, I embarked on a journey of healing and redemption. It wasn't an easy road; the scars ran deep, and the demons were relentless. But I clung to the belief that God had a purpose for me, that my pain could be transformed into something meaningful.

Through prayer, therapy, and the support of a loving community, I confronted the trauma of my past head-on. It was excruciating at times, reopening wounds that I had long buried. But as I allowed the light of God's love to penetrate the darkest corners of my soul, I began to rebuild the shattered pieces of my life.

At first, it was the simple act of surrendering to a higher power that gave me the strength to resist the allure of addiction. I leaned on my faith, finding solace in the knowledge that I was never alone in my battles. The unconditional love and forgiveness that God bestowed upon me became a guiding light, illuminating the path toward a healthier, more fulfilling life.

As I emerged from the shadows of addiction, I felt an overwhelming desire to share my newfound strength and hope with others who were still trapped in their own personal hells. I became a beacon of light, offering a helping hand to those who had lost their way. Through my own experiences, I understood their pain, their struggles, and their fears. I listened without judgment, held their hands when they trembled, and offered them a glimmer of hope when they had none.

My journey became intertwined with theirs, and together, we walked the path of recovery. We celebrated victories, no matter how small, and we mourned setbacks with compassion and understanding. Through the power of community and the unwavering love of God, we found solace in each other's stories and the knowledge that we were not alone.

As time went on, I realized that my purpose extended beyond supporting others on their journey to sobriety. I wanted to address the root causes of addiction and help prevent others from experiencing the pain and suffering I endured. I became involved in advocacy work, raising awareness about the importance of early intervention and the devastating impact of childhood trauma on addiction.

In the depths of addiction, I discovered the true power of faith, the transformative love of God, and the indomitable strength of the human spirit. Through my story, I hope to inspire others to seek help, to believe in their own capacity for change, and to embrace the unyielding light that can lead them out of the darkness. Together, we can overcome the seemingly insurmountable, and in the process, discover a life beyond addiction—a life filled with redemption, love, and unending possibilities.

As I continued my path of healing and redemption, I felt a calling deep within my soul. It was a calling to help others who were still trapped in the vicious cycle of addiction, just as I once was. I knew that my journey was not solely for my own benefit but to serve as a beacon of hope for those who felt lost and alone.

With unwavering determination, I set out to make

a difference in the lives of others. I immersed myself in volunteering at local addiction recovery centers, where I could directly connect with individuals battling their own demons. Through my own experiences, I understood their struggles, their fears, and their yearning for a way out.

I listened attentively to their stories, holding space for their pain and offering understanding without judgment. I shared my own journey, revealing the darkest moments of my past so that they could see that recovery was possible. I walked with them through the challenging steps of detoxification, withdrawal, and therapy, reminding them that they were not alone on this arduous path.

In time, I realized that my impact could reach beyond the confines of the recovery centers. I began speaking at local schools, sharing my story of addiction and resilience, with the aim of preventing young people from falling into the clutches of substance abuse. I shared the dangers of addiction and emphasized the importance of seeking help before it was too late. It was a way to give back, to use my pain as a tool for education and awareness.

Word of my journey began to spread, and I received requests to speak at conferences and events across the country. I felt a sense of responsibility to utilize these platforms to advocate for improved access to addiction treatment, mental health services, and resources for the homeless. I stood before crowds, sharing my story with unwavering vulnerability, in the hopes of inspiring change on a larger scale.

But it wasn't just about the advocacy work; it was about the connections I made along the way. Through my outreach efforts, I met individuals who shared their own stories of triumph over addiction. We formed a tight-knit community, supporting each other through the ups and downs of recovery. We celebrated milestones of sobriety, offered solace in times of relapse, and reminded each other that we were stronger together.

As my impact grew, I realized that my journey of redemption had become a lifelong commitment. I decided to pursue a career in counseling and addiction recovery, obtaining the necessary certifications and degrees to support my newfound purpose. I enrolled in psychology courses, learning the intricacies of addiction, trauma, and the power of human resilience. I knew that my firsthand experiences combined with academic knowledge would allow me to offer a unique perspective to those seeking help.

With my formal education and personal experiences, I founded a support organization for individuals in recovery. We provided a haven, offering counseling, group therapy sessions, and practical resources to help individuals rebuild their lives. It was my way of creating a space where they could find acceptance, support, and the tools needed to overcome the hurdles of addiction.

As the years went by, I witnessed countless lives

transformed through the power of faith, perseverance, and community support. I saw individuals who had hit rock bottom rise above their circumstances, discovering newfound strength and purpose. The ripple effect of their recovery extended beyond their own lives, as they, too, became advocates and mentors for others who were still on their journey to redemption.

Looking back on my own path, I am filled with gratitude for the divine intervention that guided me toward a life of healing and purpose. Every step, every struggle, and every triumph was necessary to shape me into the person I am today—a beacon of hope for those in the throes of addiction.

While the scars of my past may never fully fade, I have come to embrace them as a testament to my resilience. They serve as a constant reminder of the power of transformation and the unwavering love of God. I continue to walk alongside those who are suffering, offering them a glimmer of hope and reminding them that redemption is always within reach.

JIMMY'S STORY

I never imagined that my life could be a rollercoaster ride through hell and back. I once stood tall and proud, serving as a Marine in the war-torn landscapes of Afghanistan. But the price of my service was steep—my legs were taken from me by an IED blast, leaving me in unimaginable pain and darkness.

As a Marine, I was trained to be tough and resilient. I believed I was invincible, ready to take on any challenge thrown my way. But war has a way of stripping away illusions. It was on a dusty Afghan road that I encountered the true face of mortality. An IED explosion tore through my body, ripping away my legs and shattering the world I once knew.

In the aftermath of the blast, I was consumed by pain—both physical and emotional. The agony of losing my legs was matched only by the grief I felt for my fallen comrades. I questioned my purpose and struggled to find meaning in the face of such devastation. The darkness threatened to engulf me, and I found solace in the numbing embrace of prescription medication.

The pain of losing my legs was unbearable, but it was nothing compared to the torment that followed. I found myself drowning in a sea of despair and bitterness. The dreams I once held so dear were shattered, and a deep sense of hopelessness settled over me like a suffocating fog.

Desperate to numb both the physical and emotional pain, I turned to prescription medication. The doctors provided it to me to manage my pain, but I soon found myself relying on it as a crutch, using it to escape the harsh realities of my new reality. The pills offered a temporary respite from the constant ache, but they also brought with them a dangerous allure.

Over time, my reliance on medication morphed into a full-blown addiction. I craved the numbing effects it provided, the fleeting moments of escape from the harshness of my existence. As my dependency deepened, I lost touch with my loved ones and distanced myself from the support network that could have helped me find a way out.

Eventually, the prescriptions ran dry, and I found myself seeking solace in the darkest corners of the city. Homelessness became my reality—a bitter reminder of how far I had fallen. Days blurred into nights as I roamed the streets, desperately searching for a reprieve from the pain that plagued my body and soul.

It was in the depths of my darkest moments that I encountered a new demon—heroin. It beckoned to me like a siren, promising to silence the ghosts that tormented me. I succumbed to its grip, and it didn't take long for it to tighten its hold on my fragile existence.

My days became a relentless pursuit of the next fix, my mind consumed by the single-minded goal of numbing the pain. The streets became my home, my fellow addicts my only companions. We traded stories of desperation and loss, our lives intertwined in a web of addiction and despair.

Rock bottom hit me with a force I could never have anticipated. One fateful day, I purchased a dose of heroin that had been laced with deadly fentanyl. Unbeknownst to me, I injected the lethal cocktail into my veins. It didn't take long for the darkness to swallow me whole.

I woke up in a hospital bed, disoriented and weak. The doctors informed me that I had been in a coma for several days, my life hanging by a thread. It was a wake-up call—an opportunity for me to realize that I had been given a second chance at life.

As I lay in that hospital bed, I couldn't ignore the divine intervention that had saved me from the clutches of death. It was a stark reminder that I had a purpose—a purpose that went beyond my own pain and struggles. It was time for me to embark on a journey of redemption.

With unwavering determination, I sought help. I reached out to organizations dedicated to helping homeless veterans, and they provided me with the support and resources I desperately needed. Physical therapy became my new battleground, as I relearned how to navigate the world without my legs. It was an uphill battle, both physically and emotionally, but I refused to let my circumstances define me.

In the midst of my recovery, I discovered a beacon of hope—the unwavering love of God. I turned to prayer, seeking solace and guidance in the face of seemingly insurmountable challenges. It was through my faith that I found the strength to confront my demons head-on, to unearth the underlying issues that had led me down the treacherous path of addiction.

The road to recovery was long and filled with setbacks, but I never lost sight of the light at the end of the tunnel. I surrounded myself with a supportive community of fellow veterans, individuals who understood the unique struggles we faced. Together, we lifted each other up, offering a helping hand and a listening ear when the weight of our past threatened to consume us.

As my physical wounds healed and my sobriety solidified, I realized that my journey was not just about personal redemption—it was about paying it forward. I became passionate about helping others who were trapped in the same cycle of addiction and despair that I had once endured.

I used my own experiences as a steppingstone, sharing my story at local shelters and rehabilitation centers. I saw the spark of hope ignite in the eyes of those who had lost faith in their own recovery. I became a mentor, guiding them through the challenges and triumphs of their own journeys. I understood the battles they faced because I had fought those battles myself.

But my purpose didn't stop there. I recognized the urgent need to address the systemic issues that contributed to the cycle of addiction and homelessness among veterans. I became an advocate, lending my voice to campaigns for better access to mental health services, addiction treatment programs, and affordable housing for those who had served our country.

Today, I stand as a testament to the power of resilience and the indomitable strength of the human spirit. My past does not define me; it fuels my determination to make a positive impact on the lives of others. Each day, I strive to be a beacon of hope, a symbol that redemption is possible even in the face of unimaginable challenges.

In the depths of addiction and despair, I discovered the transformative power of faith, the resilience of the human spirit, and the infinite love of God. Through my story, I hope to inspire others to seek help, to believe in their own capacity for change, and to embrace the unyielding light that can lead them out of the darkest nights.

Together, we can overcome the seemingly insurmountable and find a life beyond addiction—a life filled with redemption, love, and unending possibilities.

ROD'S STORY

In the depths of despair, I found myself at a crossroads, believing that starting over was my only option. The idea of escaping to Cancun, a tropical paradise, beckoned to me like warm sunshine on a cold morning and offered a beacon of hope.

Haunted by a sense of rejection from my family and a failing marriage, I saw Cancun as a chance for a clean slate. As an entrepreneur with a travel business background and fluency in Spanish, it seemed like a logical choice. The allure of white sandy beaches, turquoise waters, and the opportunity to sell timeshares enticed me. Perhaps I could even find a treatment center to overcome my addictions and start afresh in a marketing position.

Driven by the prospect of a fresh start, I impulsively booked a one-way ticket. Without a word to anyone, I embarked on a journey that would forever alter the course of my life.

As I traveled toward Cancun, doubts began to cloud my mind. A layover in Denver became a turning point, where conflicting thoughts overwhelmed me. Questions about money, withdrawal symptoms, and the uncertainty of my future in Cancun cast a shadow over my grand plans. I realized that escape might not be the solution I desperately sought.

Reflecting on my life, I came from a privileged background, enjoying the luxuries of a loving family and entrepreneurial success. However, I succumbed to the temptations of a wilder lifestyle. Alcohol became my elixir, and the introduction of an addictive substance called GHB sparked my downward spiral. My addiction wreaked havoc on my personal and professional life, leaving me estranged from my wife and desperate for a way out.

The journey of self-discovery is a profound one and experience is often our greatest teacher. Unbeknownst to me, that first sip of GHB led to a twenty-year battle with addiction, resulting in sleepless nights, DUIs, jail sentences, and devastating losses. It stripped me of everything, including pride, businesses, finances, homes, cars, and cherished relationships. My wife saw me transform into a different person, often referring to me as Dr. Jekyll and Mr. Hyde, questioning where the good man she married had gone.

Homeless, without a car or job, I sought refuge in a friend's spare bedroom while selling Bitcoin mining. However, when caught smoking crack in his house, I was forced to find a cheap hotel, feeling utterly alone. In this desperate state, I hatched a plan to escape to Cancun.

Life hinges on critical split-second decisions that can shape our destiny. Realizing this, I chose to redefine

F.E.A.R. from "Forget Everything And Run" to "Face Everything And Rise" and return home. Uncertain if my friend would accept me back, I called him, pouring out my betrayal and despair. Despite his disappointment, he lifted me up, reminding me of a time when I offered him hope in his darkest moment. Now, our roles were reversed, and he encouraged me to reach out to God.

In that pivotal moment, my friend bore witness to the possibility of God freeing me from the demon of addiction. Urging me to call out with unwavering faith, he assured me that God, the Creator, had the power to grant my plea. Exhausted and ready for change, I cried out to my Creator, surrendering completely and asking for release from my obsessive cravings. That night, an indescribable sense of calm and peace washed over me, leaving me sobbing with happiness and an overwhelming feeling of love and hope. God spoke to my soul, assuring me that everything would be alright and revealing that my pain had a purpose in His perfect plan.

In a twist of fate, my probation officer appeared at my door, not to arrest me but to provide an opportunity for rehabilitation. Encouraged by this unexpected turn, I found myself at The Retreat at ZION, a residential rehab center near the awe-inspiring ZION National Park. The owner, Robert "Cord" Beatty, had faced his own battles with addiction and offered a guiding light on my path to recovery.

Immersed in the healing process, I discovered the power of self-reflection and the beauty of nature. The canyons of ZION became my sanctuary, where I communed with God and confronted the demons within. The journey was not easy, but each step brought me closer to understanding my purpose.

Looking back, I recognized that destiny is not merely a matter of chance but a product of the choices we make. My impulsive decision to escape to Cancun led me on a journey of self-discovery and redemption. Today, I stand as a testament to the power of faith, surrender, and the capacity for change.

My story is not one of regret but of gratitude. It is a testament to the transformative power of embracing pain and finding the strength to rise above it. With unwavering determination, I continue to walk this path, inspiring others to embrace their own personal journeys of healing and growth.

Through my own experiences, I have come to understand the profound impact of addiction on individuals and their loved ones. It is a disease that knows no boundaries, affecting people from all walks of life. However, I firmly believe that recovery is possible for everyone, and it begins with a willingness to confront one's demons and embark on a path of self-discovery.

For me, this journey has been more than just personal redemption. It has been an opportunity to connect with others, to share my story, and to inspire hope in those who may feel lost or trapped by addiction. I have witnessed countless lives transformed, individuals who have reclaimed their dignity, rebuilt their relationships, and discovered a newfound sense of purpose.

As I reflect on my tumultuous past, I am filled with gratitude for every twist and turn that led me to this point. My struggles were not in vain but served as steppingstones toward a higher purpose. Today, I am humbled to be able to guide others toward the path of recovery, offering them the same hope and support that was extended to me.

If you or someone you know is battling addiction, know that you are not alone. There is a community ready to embrace you, support you, and guide you toward a brighter future.

Remember, within every story of pain lies the potential for remarkable resilience and growth. Embrace your journey, trust in the power to change, and discover the strength within you to rise above your circumstances. The road to recovery may be challenging, but it is a journey well worth taking.

CANDICE'S STORY

My life's journey has been marked by a series of traumas that tested my spirit and shattered my sense of self-worth. But through it all, I have discovered the transformative power of God's love and redemption.

I was born in the vibrant city of Las Vegas in 1984, the youngest of three girls. My earliest childhood memory is of Easter morning at the tender age of five. My parents' heated argument escalated, and in a fit of anger, my mother hurled a frozen cornish hen at my father, narrowly missing him. Even at such a young age, I could feel the tension and hostility in my home, setting the stage for years of turmoil to come.

Around the same time, my innocence was stolen when I became the victim of inappropriate touching by a family member. Fearful of causing trouble, I kept this dark secret hidden, locking away the pain and shame deep within my heart. Tragically, this same family member's child began to touch me inappropriately, continuing the cycle of abuse for years to come.

At the age of seven, my parents' marriage crumbled under the weight of my mother's multiple affairs, resulting in their divorce. Both of my parents went on to marry multiple times, bringing instability and confusion into our lives. My mother's hurtful words and constant blame towards me left me feeling like a burden and a mistake. As she remarried, her new husband introduced me to cigarettes and alcohol at a tender age, leaving me vulnerable and susceptible to the darkness that loomed ahead.

But what was even more disturbing was his unsettling behavior, such as watching my sisters and me while we slept. When I mustered the courage to share my concerns with my mother, she dismissed me, accusing me of trying to ruin her marriage. Feeling abandoned and unimportant, I learned to keep my pain and fears locked away, believing that no one would listen or understand.

At the age of ten, my world was shattered once again when my best friend from school was brutally murdered by her brother during a visit to California. The weight of grief and loss was almost too much to bear, and I struggled to cope with the emotional turmoil that ensued. I couldn't shake the guilt of not being there with her that fateful weekend, as my father had forbidden me from going.

Recognizing the impact of my friend's death on my behavior, my father decided to take me and my middle sister into his full-time care. My mother didn't fight this decision, leaving me feeling abandoned once again. My father did his best to provide a happy family environment, taking us to church and trying to be there for us. But my deep-seated anger towards my mother and my perception of God as someone who had taken my best friend away, made me a ticking time bomb, filled with resentment and frustration.

At the age of thirteen, I became sexually active at fourteen, using it as a temporary escape from the pain I felt inside. I engaged in risky behaviors, meeting strangers from the internet, and engaging in promiscuity. My life was filled with anger and self-destructive patterns.

My father remarried, but the new woman in his life treated me poorly, and I felt like an outcast in my own home. Seeking solace, I worked three jobs while attending school to escape the tense environment. At eighteen, I entered a verbally and physically abusive relationship with a much older man, further fueling my downward spiral.

Despite my chaotic lifestyle, I enrolled in the police academy, hoping marriage and starting a family would bring stability to my life. However, I married impulsively at twenty-three, only to find myself in another toxic relationship that led to infidelity and more pain. The abuse escalated, and I lived in constant fear.

As a police officer, I faced the harsh realities of life daily, witnessing tragic deaths and experiencing traumatic events. I suppressed my emotions, becoming hardened and unfeeling, hiding behind a facade of strength. The culture of policing discouraged talking about feelings, reinforcing my inability to process the traumatic experiences I encountered.

Amidst the darkness, a glimmer of hope appeared in my life. I met Michael, a man who offered responsibility, stability, and a loving family. Despite some warning signs, I overlooked them, longing for a sense of security. We married, but the shadows of my past continued to haunt me. In January of 2015, Michael's choices led to his arrest, and in that moment of despair, I turned to God in prayer. He whispered to my heart, urging me to stay and witness the miracle He had planned for our family. Michael's arrest marked a turning point in both our lives. He quit drinking, and I joined him in giving up alcohol. This decision forced me to confront the pain I had numbed with alcohol for so long.

With newfound determination, I sought help from a Christ-centered program that proved to be transformative. Attending their Step Study, I confronted my past, acknowledging my brokenness and embracing God's love and forgiveness. My heart began to heal, and I found solace in the verse, Jeremiah 29:11, realizing that God had plans for my life, plans filled with hope and a future.

As I progressed in my recovery, I felt a calling to share my story and help others find healing through the 12 steps. I began serving as a leader in the program, witnessing firsthand the transformative power of God's love in the lives of others.

The journey was not without challenges. I faced the passing of my mother, but instead of turning to alcohol, I leaned on the tools I had acquired, allowing me to process my grief and forgive her before she passed.

Despite making great strides, life had one more hurdle for me. In June of 2020, the stress of my work as a sexual assault detective and unresolved traumas led to intrusive thoughts of suicide. Seeking help, I was diagnosed with PTSD, depression, and anxiety, and I made the difficult decision to medically retire from the police force.

Through it all, my recovery group remained a safe space where I could be vulnerable and find acceptance and support. My faith in God deepened, and I embraced the principle of submission to God's will, understanding that my weaknesses could be turned into strengths through Him.

Today, I stand as a living testament to God's grace and love, a testimony of hope and healing for others who are still lost in the darkness. No longer a victim, I have found redemption and restoration through God's mercy and grace. Through my recovery group, I have discovered a community that has helped me find healing and purpose in my life.

To anyone who feels burdened by their past, I implore you to seek help, to reach out to God, and to find a community of support. My life is a testament to the fact that God's love is boundless, His grace is sufficient, and His power is transformative. Embrace the journey of healing, and let God's love lead you to a place of freedom, joy, and restoration.

My prayer is that sharing my story with others will serve as a reminder that no matter how broken or lost we may feel, God's love has the power to heal, restore, and redeem every broken piece of our lives. May His grace guide you, His love sustains you, and His peace envelop you as you embark on your own journey of healing and redemption.

MARSHA'S STORY

My earliest memories were in Delores, Colorado, when I was 5 years old. We lived in a beautiful farm-style home on a quiet street, just 1 ½ blocks from the rushing Animus river. Delores was a small town of about 1000 people at the time. My dad worked for the US Forest Service and was a firefighter. As a bold little girl with a mind of my own, I did whatever I wanted and didn't listen to my mother much. She rarely tried to restrain me.

I remember one Sunday morning when I was particularly adventurous. I got dressed for church and told my mom I was going. Despite being only five years old and having never been to church before, I was determined to go. Surprisingly, my mom didn't stop me, and I happily skipped and ran, hoping not to be late. I ended up in the Catholic Church down the street, fascinated by the ritualistic nature of the service, even though I didn't understand the language.

After church, I went to the Baptist Church across the street, drawn by the singing. I pretended to belong there and even told someone I would come back to Sunday school the next week. I continued attending the Baptist church and tried to share my newfound love for church with my parents, but they didn't pay much attention. So, I would retreat to the backyard, sit under a tree, and tell my leprechaun all about it.

Unfortunately, my family life wasn't as joyful as my church experiences. My parents constantly fought, yelling and saying hurtful things to each other. I would hide behind a door, crying, and hold my little brother Eddie close. Sometimes, after their fights, I would go out and cry to my leprechaun, but my little brother couldn't see him and thought I was just playing.

I loved learning about God and Jesus, and my fascination with the church grew stronger. My parents never talked to me about God, but my mom would sometimes say, "Honey, everything is going to be alright." Despite the chaos at home, I remained outgoing and unafraid of talking to strangers. I would share random facts like the alphabet and the states and their capitals with anyone who would listen.

My early years were marked by a family structure steeped in alcoholism and addiction. I was born in Durango, Colorado, one of five children at the time. My parents and all of my siblings, except one, struggled with addiction due to our genetic makeup.

We lived a nomadic lifestyle, living in our car from the time I was five to eleven years old. My dad lost his job due to his drinking, and my mother's drinking habits worsened. At times, she would leave my brother and me with relatives while she went off to drink and engage in questionable activities.

During these years, I experienced sexual abuse by a cousin, and I carried this secret inside me for a long time. We lived in poverty, begging for food and drinking water from ponds. My brother and I were constantly alone, our education neglected. I tried to teach him, but he had little interest in learning.

One day, my grandparents rescued us from the chaos. I lived with them for a couple of years, feeling loved and cared for. Still, the guilt and resentment towards my parents and my little brother lingered, and I struggled with self-harm as a way to cope with my pain.

Eventually, my mother convinced my grandparents to give her another chance to take care of me. Reluctantly, I went back to live with her, hoping things might be different. However, her promises were short-lived, and the chaotic lifestyle resumed. She would leave us for weeks at a time, leaving my brother and me fending for ourselves.

At the age of 12, I refused to get into her car one last time, deciding to leave my little brother behind to ensure my own survival. I sought refuge with the Stafford family, friends who welcomed me into their home. My life improved significantly under their care, and I felt loved and accepted.

In college, my life took a downward turn as I began using alcohol and drugs to cope with my past. I eventually dropped out of school and moved with my boyfriend

Denton to Salt Lake City to help care for his father. We got married to please his father, but it wasn't the fairy tale I had hoped for.

My husband Denton and I were deeply in love and enjoyed being married, but a significant issue arose over the years - we both became functional alcoholic/addicts. Despite having good jobs, material possessions, and a home, our lives revolved around drinking and using drugs to cope with our problems. We also became workaholics, with my job at Holiday Inn allowing me to drink with customers while I worked.

Throughout my career, I climbed the corporate ladder, starting as a waitress and eventually becoming a General Manager. After ten years in the hotel industry, I shifted to the Food Distribution industry for the next decade. However, my addiction took a toll on my mental health, leading to drug-induced psychosis and a loss of reality.

In 1997, I had a profound experience that made me realize my disease was progressing rapidly. My mental state deteriorated to the point where I could no longer distinguish between reality and delusions. At a low point, I attempted suicide by driving my car off a cliff. Thankfully, I survived and encountered a comforting presence that I believed to be Jesus.

Despite this event, I continued to struggle with addiction and alcoholism for the next three years, leading to the complete ruin of my life. I was financially bankrupt, had isolated myself from family, and my relationship with my husband was deeply strained due to our codependent drug use. I had lost my job and my self-image, believing my identity was solely tied to my job title.

Eventually, I hit rock bottom and realized I needed help. On March 11th, 2000, I made the decision to save my life and seek the assistance I desperately needed. I was an addict and an alcoholic, and my actions had led to severe consequences, including a ten-year prison sentence. I was emotionally and physically broken, but with the realization that I had reached my lowest point, I was motivated to seek treatment.

My journey of recovery began when I humbly asked for help and sought therapy. Despite my difficult past, I embraced the chance to change my life. Through therapy and Alcoholics Anonymous, I found the strength to rebuild my life and pursue a career in counseling. I became an entrepreneur and founded a non-profit organization, New U Recovery, to help others struggling with addiction.

Along the way, I faced challenges, including a difficult decision to divorce my husband due to his return to drug and alcohol use. But I stayed true to my sobriety and focused on my purpose to help others recover. With faith in God's guidance, I opened sober living houses and engaged in various projects to promote recovery.

I continue to grow, learning and pursuing education to enhance my abilities as a counselor and storyteller. My vision for the future involves carrying the message of hope and recovery while exploring the world and its adventures.

Through it all, I aim to inspire others to grow where they are planted and spread the beauty of hope and love wherever they go.

I found myself at the beginning of a remarkable journey that led me to this beautiful place, where I can now share a part of my story of recovery. There was a time when I felt humbled enough to ask for help and make an appointment with a therapist. I remember vividly sitting outside that facility, pondering my choices - should I stay and face my struggles or should I run away from them? Tears streamed down my face as I realized I had to make a critical decision: either save myself or surrender to the darkness that was consuming me.

Summoning every ounce of strength within me, I took a deep breath and stepped through the doors of that facility, the doors that would open the path to the rest of my life. Sitting with the therapist, I felt like a faucet had been turned on as she asked me to share my story, something no one had ever done before. How could it take 41 years for someone to care enough to ask about me?

I shared my story, a painful tale of suffering from alcohol, drugs, and sexual abuse. In my heart, I knew it wasn't my fault; anyone would have turned to substances in the face of such pain. Yet, in that moment, I felt like a defeated soldier, battered by life's blows. Little did

I know that this therapist would be the catalyst for my transformation, inspiring me to pursue a career as a counselor to help others as she had helped me.

She offered me an Intensive Outpatient (IOP) treatment and introduced me to Alcoholics Anonymous (AA). I hesitated at first, but I chose to embrace the help she was offering me. Memories of my grandfather, who had been my hero and a pillar of strength with 30 years of sobriety in AA, resurfaced. His words and the serenity prayer hanging on his wall had left a lasting impact on me. With this newfound hope, I attended my first meeting at the Alano Club, and it felt like home.

With the tools I gained in recovery, I became a changed person, with new friends, new hope, and a new attitude. Someone believed in me enough to support my Alcohol and Drug Counseling program at the University of Utah, where I eventually became a counselor and a probation officer. These individuals became my new heroes, guiding me in my journey.

Throughout my life, I have always sought heroes to show me the way, to provide something or someone to believe in when life seemed bleak. As I graduated from college and spoke at the ceremony, I encouraged my classmates to rise up and help others find their way out of the darkness of addiction and discover their true selves.

In the initial five years of sobriety, the Big Book of Alcoholics Anonymous came alive for me, becoming a blueprint for my life. I worked the steps, they worked me, and then I lived the steps, resulting in a profound connection with my higher power, God.

The following ten years of my recovery were a journey of discovery and spiritual growth. I embraced a path of awakening and purification of the mind, gradually progressing towards enlightenment and a unitive life, a journey that spans a lifetime.

My life took a turn when I embarked on a new endeavor to establish a non-profit treatment center to help those struggling with addiction. Through a series of events, I met Cord, a friend and supporter who helped make my dream a reality. With his assistance, I founded New U Recovery Inc., connecting people and families affected by addiction to the services they need.

Despite facing personal challenges, including the end of my marriage due to my husband's return to addiction, I held onto my sobriety and my faith in God. His guidance and support led me to open the first Sober Living House in St. George, Utah.

As my journey continued, I found myself co-hosting a recovery radio show, producing a documentary, and writing a book, all aimed at giving back to the recovery community and inspiring others on their paths to healing.

One of the greatest experiences of my journey in recovery has been watching my family overcome the pain and suffering of addiction. All of my siblings are sober

My oldest brother was released from prison 7 years ago and has maintained his sobriety My sister Debbie was the last to get sober and she is 67 got sober 3 years ago My mom is a miracle in my family she got sober at the age of 87 she's now 92 a vibrant and wonderful amazing woman who knows God and credits him for her sobriety and her children sobriety we are blessed as a family under God's watchful care

My journey is a testament to the power of resilience, faith, and self-discovery. From the depths of addiction to the heights of recovery and purpose, I have learned to trust in a higher power and to serve others on their journey to wholeness. My life's purpose is clear - to be a tool for God, helping those in need and sharing the gift of recovery.

AMY'S STORY

As I sit down to pen my story, the memories of my lost innocence flood my mind, transporting me back to that fateful day when my world shattered into a million broken pieces. I was a bright-eyed, hopeful young girl, unaware of the darkness that lurked in the shadows of the world.

It started as an ordinary day, with the laughter of children echoing through the neighborhood and the warmth of the sun casting its gentle glow. Little did I know that this façade of normalcy would soon be shattered, leaving me exposed and vulnerable to the evils that lay in wait.

As the sun began its descent, signaling the approach of twilight, I found myself walking alone along a quiet street. In the blink of an eye, a vehicle screeched to a halt beside me, its menacing presence filling the air. Fear instantly coursed through my veins, paralyzing me with a terror I had never experienced before.

Before I could comprehend what was happening, I was forcibly dragged into the depths of the vehicle, the sound of my screams drowned out by the deafening silence of my captors. They were cold and ruthless, devoid of any trace of humanity. It was then that I realized the magnitude of the nightmare I had unwittingly stumbled into.

Days turned into weeks, and weeks into months, as I was transported to a desolate place far away from the life I once knew. It was there that I was thrown into a web of despair and darkness, surrounded by others who shared my fate. We became nothing more than commodities, stripped of our identities and reduced to mere objects to be bought and sold.

The horrors I endured were beyond comprehension, etching deep scars on my body and soul. The physical abuse was excruciating, leaving me battered and bruised, while the emotional torment eroded the very essence of my being. Every day was a battle to survive, to find a sliver of hope amid the pervasive darkness that threatened to consume me.

The traumas I endured left me with a void, an emptiness that begged to be filled. Seeking solace, I sought refuge in substances that promised temporary relief, an escape from the torment that plagued my every waking moment. A way to numb the pain, to forget, if only for a little while. But addiction has a cunning way of taking hold, sinking its hooks into the vulnerable spaces within us. The substances that once provided solace soon became my captors, ensnaring me in a vicious cycle of dependency.

Days turned into nights, and nights into a blur of self-destructive behaviors. The grip of addiction tightened around me, squeezing the life out of my fragile existence. I became a slave to the very substances that were meant to liberate me from my pain.

The world outside became a distant memory as my world shrank to the confines of my addiction. Relationships crumbled, opportunities slipped through my fingers, and my dreams were suffocated by the weight of my dependency. I was consumed by shame and guilt, unable to recognize the person I had become.

Physical withdrawal symptoms wreaked havoc on my already battered body, while the psychological cravings gnawed at my sanity. Desperation replaced the glimmer of hope that had once flickered within me. The abyss of addiction seemed bottomless, and I found myself teetering on the precipice of despair. A profound realization that my addiction had now made me prisoner of my reality. It was here that I would survive and ultimately find my death.

In the midst of my darkest hour, a flicker of hope ignited within me. It was a seemingly chance encounter with a stranger, a compassionate soul who spoke words that resonated deep within my broken spirit. He told me of a power greater than myself, a force of love and redemption that could lift me from the depths of my despair.

It was through his guidance that I began to open my heart to the possibility of a connection with God. Through prayer, meditation, and surrender, I found solace in the arms of the divine. It was in this newfound relationship that I discovered the strength to confront my demons and embark on a path of healing. It was in deed the strength I needed to leave this life and start over.

Recovery was not an easy road. It demanded unwavering commitment and a willingness to face the pain I had long suppressed. With the support of fellow survivors and mentors who understood my journey, I slowly started to rebuild my life.

Therapy sessions, support groups, and the unwavering presence of God became my guiding lights. With every step forward, I shed the shackles of addiction, reclaiming my identity and discovering a strength I never knew existed within me.

Today, I stand as a testament to the power of resilience and faith. No longer defined by my past, I have dedicated my life to helping others who are trapped in the clutches of addiction. Child abduction, and sex trafficking. I have become a voice for the voiceless, a beacon of hope for those still lost in the darkness.

Through my own experiences, I empathize with their struggles, offering guidance and support as they navigate their own paths to recovery. Together, we confront the demons that once haunted us, knowing that we are not alone in our battles.

As I reflect on my journey, I am humbled by the transformation that has taken place within me. From a shattered young girl to a survivor, I have emerged stronger than ever before. It is through my connection with God that I have found redemption and purpose.

My story serves as a testament to the indomitable spirit of the human soul. No matter how deep the darkness, there is always a glimmer of light waiting to be discovered. May my journey inspire others to seek solace, find strength in their faith, and overcome the most formidable of challenges.

In sharing my story, I hope to ignite the flicker of hope within those who are still trapped in the grip of addiction. Together, we can forge a path towards healing, and in doing so, discover the transformative power of God's love.

RANDY'S STORY

I was just a young boy when I first laid eyes on a professional pilot soaring through the skies. The gleaming cockpit and the mesmerizing view from above left an indelible mark on my impressionable mind. From that moment, I knew what I wanted to be when I grew up - an airline pilot, traveling the world and experiencing the freedom of flight.

As the years passed, I dedicated my life to achieving that dream. I studied hard, worked tirelessly, and earned my wings. Becoming a pilot fulfilled me in ways I could have never imagined. The thrill of taking off, the sense of responsibility, and the camaraderie with my fellow crew members gave me a profound sense of purpose.

But as the years rolled on, the rigors of the job began to take their toll. Long flights, irregular sleep patterns, and the constant pressure to perform at the highest level weighed heavily on my shoulders. I was no stranger to stress, but I was unprepared for the emotional rollercoaster that awaited me.

On overnight flights, loneliness and fatigue often gripped me. I found myself seeking solace in alcohol to cope with the anxieties that came with each flight. A drink here and there became a ritual, helping me unwind and escape the pressures of the job. It seemed harmless at first, but little did I know that it would soon lead me down a treacherous path.

As time went on, those occasional drinks turned into a habit, and soon, I was relying on alcohol to numb the anxieties that were creeping into my life. The stress of flying combined with the weight of personal problems created a perfect storm of addiction.

Many times, I would find myself flying while hungover or with the lingering effects of alcohol in my system. Sometimes, I would have a shot or two from the mini bottles in my hotel room prior to going to work. It was a desperate attempt to stop the shakes and the anxiety that threatened to consume me. The guilt and shame gnawed at my conscience, but addiction had ensnared me in its relentless grip.

I was a master at hiding my addiction, or so I thought. I would show up to work with a forced smile and a mask of strength, but deep down, I was falling apart. My performance as a pilot started to suffer, and I struggled to maintain the level of excellence expected of me. The pressures of the job coupled with my secret battle became a heavy burden to bear.

It was only a matter of time before my secret was exposed. One fateful day, I failed an alcohol test.

My world came crashing down around me as the consequences of my actions came to light. I was suspended from my position as a pilot, pending an investigation. I was devastated, and the reality of what I had become hit me like a ton of bricks.

I faced disciplinary hearings and the uncertainty of my future in aviation. My career, the very thing that had defined me, was now hanging in the balance. The shame and guilt were suffocating, and I was left to confront the wreckage of my life. I felt like I had let down not only myself but also my loved ones, who had always believed in me.

As the days turned into weeks, the uncertainty gnawed at me, and the weight of my actions became unbearable. My marriage, once a pillar of strength, began to crumble under the weight of my addiction. My wife, a woman of unwavering support, watched helplessly as her husband spiraled out of control.

The day came when I received the news I had been dreading. I had lost my license and my career as an airline pilot. The consequences of my addiction were finally catching up with me, and I had no one to blame but myself.

With the financial pressure and my alcoholism out of control, my wife had no other choice but to leave me and protect our children. My world crumbled. I began to loose everything including my home, and assets. With my career in shambles, my marriage in ruins, and my future uncertain, I hit rock bottom. I found myself homeless, wandering the streets with nothing but the clothes on my back and the weight of my failures on my shoulders. I slept in cheap hotels and stayed with friends who would take me in until my drinking destroyed those relationships.

In the darkness of my despair, a glimmer of hope emerged. A fellow recovering alcoholic, a stranger who had once walked in my shoes, reached out to me. He offered to take me through the 12 steps, and in that moment, I saw a lifeline - a chance to find redemption. It was an divine intervention and moment of clarity that I so desperately needed. With nothing left to lose, I decided to embrace this lifeline. I embarked on the arduous journey of the 12 steps, confronting the demons of my past and the pain I had caused. Each step brought me closer to a power greater than myself, a spiritual awakening that I had never experienced before.

Through the steps, I accepted my addiction and surrendered myself to God, seeking guidance and strength to navigate the turbulent waters of sobriety. It was not an easy journey, and I faced moments of doubt and uncertainty. But each day of sobriety became a victory, and I clung to the newfound hope that was rekindled within me.

As I trudged through the steps, I also began to mend the broken pieces of my life. I sought reconciliation with my wife. With humility and honesty, I laid bare my struggles and sought her forgiveness. Miraculously, she embraced me with love and compassion. She saw the effort I was putting into my recovery and decided to give our marriage another chance. It was a turning point in our lives, a second chance at rebuilding our life together. Suddenly, my once coveted career didn't matter any longer.

Through my journey of redemption, I discovered a new purpose - to be an advocate, teacher, and mentor to young men who struggled with alcohol. I shared my story, my struggles, and my transformation to show them that there is a way out of the darkness.

With each person I helped, I found healing for my own wounds. I realized that my journey was not just about my own recovery but about making a difference in the lives of others. I became a voice for those who felt lost and alone, offering them hope and a path to redemption.

Today, I stand as a testament to the power of recovery and the strength of the human spirit. Sobriety has given me a clarity of mind and a sense of purpose that I had never known before. I wake up every day grateful for the gift of redemption and the opportunity to help others find their way.

My journey is far from over, and I still carry the scars of my past. But I wear them with pride, for they are a reminder of the battles I have fought and the victory I have achieved. Each day, I walk with a renewed sense of purpose, knowing that my story can be a beacon of hope for those who are lost in the depths of addiction.

Life is now filled with meaning and purpose, and I am forever indebted to that stranger who offered me a lifeline in my darkest hour. Their act of kindness set me on the path to redemption, and it is a path I am proud to walk every day. I am not defined by my past mistakes; I am defined by my resilience and the transformation that came from embracing recovery. Today, I am not just a pilot, but a man on a mission to make a difference in the lives of others. Through my own experiences, I have come to understand the power of compassion, empathy, and support in the journey to recovery. I strive to be a beacon of hope for those who have lost their way, just as someone once was for me.

As an advocate and mentor, I work closely with organizations that focus on addiction recovery. I share my story at seminars, workshops, and support groups, offering a message of hope and resilience. I want those who are struggling to know that they are not alone and that there is a community of people who care and understand. My advocacy work also extends to pilots within the aviation industry. I collaborate with airlines and aviation organizations to raise awareness about the dangers of substance abuse and the importance of mental health support for pilots. The aviation industry is highly regulated, but we must continue to ensure that there is a supportive environment for pilots to seek help when needed. Through my efforts, I've seen a positive change in the aviation community's approach to mental health and addiction. More pilots are coming forward to seek help without fear of judgment or stigma. We have set up confidential support networks and counseling services, offering a lifeline to those who may be struggling.

As my journey of redemption continues, I've also made it a personal mission to rebuild the relationships that were fractured by my addiction. With the support of my wife, we attended counseling together, taking the necessary steps to heal and nurture our marriage.

It wasn't an easy road, and there were moments of doubt and pain, but our commitment to each other and the newfound strength from my recovery allowed us to rebuild trust and create a stronger foundation for our future together.

Today, we are closer than ever before, and I am grateful for her unwavering love and support. We cherish each day, knowing that our love and commitment have weathered the storm of addiction and emerged stronger than ever.

My journey has taught me the importance of surrendering to a higher power, and I now walk hand-in-hand with God, finding solace in my faith. It is through this spiritual awakening that I have discovered inner peace and a sense of purpose.

I stand before you today, not as a fallen pilot, but as a man who has risen from the ashes of addiction and found a higher purpose. My life's journey is now dedicated to helping others find their way, just as someone once did for me.

As I take to the skies once more, it is not just the aircraft that carries me, but the wings of redemption, hope, and resilience. My journey continues, and I am committed to soaring higher, shining brighter, and making a difference in the lives of those who need it most.

Through the gift of redemption, I have discovered a new flight path - one that leads to a destination of hope, healing, and the boundless possibilities of a life free from addiction. And with each new day, I embrace this journey with gratitude, knowing that my story can be a lifeline for those who are seeking theirs.

TIFFANIE'S STORY

In a world filled with trials and tribulations, mine started around the age of 6. I endured tremendous hardships and experienced traumas that left deep scars on my heart. The loss of her beloved brother shattered my innocence, and the weight of grief and sorrow followed me like a shadow. Shortly after his death, I began to be sexually violated and that violation lasted for years.

As I grew older, the pain manifested in different ways, leading me to struggle with eating disorders, major depression, and crippling anxiety. In my search for happiness and belonging, I found myself in a toxic marriage that spanned fifteen years. The love I had hoped for turned into a prison of emotional torment, leaving me feeling trapped and isolated.

Despite the darkness that engulfed my life, I held onto a glimmer of hope. I knew deep down that there had to be a way to heal and find peace within myself. The universe heard my prayers, and a spark of fate intervened when I met a kind and understanding soul who would become my savior.

I remarried, and as my new husband and I embarked on the journey of starting a family, we experienced a traumatic miscarriage. The pain of loss was indescribable, and I found myself sinking further into despair. My emotional wounds were ripped open once more, and I struggled to cope with the heartbreak.

Finally, after a difficult pregnancy, I gave birth to a beautiful, healthy, perfect baby girl. However, the joy of motherhood was overshadowed by postpartum anxiety and depression, making it difficult for me to find solace in the love I had for my miracle baby.

Feeling like I had reached the end of my rope, I decided to seek professional help one last time. I hoped that this therapist would be the one to guide me towards real healing and renewal. I had completely given up at this point. I felt suicidal and had told my family that I was prepared to die that day. Unfortunately, this encounter turned out to be yet another triggering experience, pushing me to the brink of giving up forever.

But within the depths of despair, I sat in the parking lot of the clinic and found the strength to utter one last prayer. I pleaded for a beacon of light to guide me out of the darkness that had consumed my life for so long.

Miraculously, my prayer was answered. I opened my phone seeking someone, somewhere and as if guided by an unseen force, I stumbled upon the Zion Healing Center. This place, with its warm and compassionate environment, felt like a sanctuary of hope and possibility. The caring staff at the center embraced me with open arms, understanding the depths of my pain without judgment.

Through a combination of therapy, support, and holistic healing techniques, I began to mend my broken spirit. I learned to embrace my past, acknowledging that my journey of healing was nonlinear but worth every step.

With time, love, and patience, my wounds began to heal, and I emerged from the shadows as a new person. The process was not without setbacks, but each time I stumbled, I found strength in the supportive community at the Zion Healing Center.

My life transformed in more ways than I could have imagined. Filled with gratitude for the newfound hope and second chance, I decided to dedicate my life to helping others who were once in my shoes.

I joined the Zion Healing Center, drawing from my personal experiences to connect with those seeking solace. My journey of healing gave me the empathy and compassion needed to guide others towards their own path of renewal. As I share my story and listened to the stories of others, I witness the power of hope and the resilience of the human spirit. Together with the team at the center, I try to help give new hope and new life to others, just as they had done for me.

My journey was not easy, but I embraced it with newfound strength and grace. I had walked through the darkness and found my way to the other side, shining like a beacon of hope for those still lost in the shadows.

And so, the woman who once said her goodbyes to the world found purpose and new life through the healing power of love and support. My life became a testament to the fact that even in the depths of despair, there is always a glimmer of hope, waiting to be discovered.

MATT'S STORY

In the unforgiving grip of fate, I found myself hurtling down a path I never envisioned, an addict ensnared by opiates. It's a tragic truth that no one sets out to become an addict, and my tale of addiction to these sinister substances is no exception.

January 16, 2006, marks the fateful day when my world was shattered in a violent, life-altering car accident. The brutal impact left me paralyzed from the waist down, a mere 30 years old, robbed of my mobility and independence. My body, once whole and vibrant, now bore the scars of a relentless battle. Not one, but two surgeries left my spine fused from shoulder blades to lumbar spine, trapping me in a prison of agony.

Oh, the pain, it was unrelenting and merciless, like a malevolent specter haunting my every moment. My body became a stranger, and fear gripped my soul, taunting me with the prospect of a future without hope. All I yearned for was to reclaim the freedom to walk, to move, to be whole once more.

With fierce determination, I defied medical expectations, surpassing the boundaries of possibility. I pushed myself beyond human limits, achieving what was deemed impossible in the sterile confines of hospital charts. Yet, for every victory won, I paid a steep price: suffering, torment, and endless torment.

In this dance with darkness, a sinister temptress named OxyContin appeared, a seductive mirage of relief. Oblivious to its treacherous allure, I swallowed the pill of false hope. Lo and behold, I found myself pushing through therapies with newfound vigor, my shattered body momentarily liberated from its shackles of agony.

Within the hallowed halls of LDS Hospital in Salt Lake City, Utah, I toiled to relearn life's most basic tasks—sitting up, rolling over, showering, and dressing myself. But it was not mere strength or courage that propelled me; it was the deceptive embrace of OxyContin that masked my pain.

Dismissed from the hospital's care, I carried with me the devilish concoction, OxyContin 10 mg, prescribed for my "long-term pain," and Lortab 10 mg to contend with moments of unbearable agony. Unable to silence the relentless screams of pain that gnawed at me, clawing away my will to endure. In desperation, I confessed my plight to the doctors and therapists, my pleas resonating through the sterile walls of the medical domain. And so it was agreed upon to increase my dosage. OxyContin rose to 30 mg, and Lortab yielded to the might of two Percocet 10 mg.

A deceptive dance played out, as the drugs allowed me to push my frail body to achieve the impossible once more. With sheer determination, I rose from the abyss of paralysis, embracing the liberation of walking once again, aided by a walker. But the euphoria of triumph was fleeting, replaced by the crushing reality that my newfound strength was merely an illusion, crafted by the numbing haze of addiction.

In the darkest depths of my opiate entanglement, I found myself at the summit of abuse, consuming a staggering trio of OxyContin 80s each day, one with the morning sun, another right after my grueling therapy sessions in the afternoon, and the final one before surrendering to the night's embrace. But even this relentless regimen couldn't satiate my insatiable hunger for relief. I was entangled in the clutches of Roxycontin, a pure opiate devoid of Tylenol, a cruel necessity due to my ailing kidneys, tormented by the presence of Tylenol in Percocet. A prisoner to my pain, I swallowed 480 pills every fortnight, a staggering 390 mg of opiate coursing through my veins daily.

My descent into addiction wasn't paved with heedless indulgence in recreational drugs; no, it began innocently, with a justifiable need to ease my suffering, prescribed these potent medications as my lifeline. Endless days melted into five long years of relentless therapy, a ceaseless cycle, seven days a week, all for the elusive hope of walking again. But the cruel hands of fate refused to release me from my wheelchair's iron grip, leaving me bitter and disillusioned.

My once robust back now played host to an intricate fusion of titanium rods, screws, a plate, and a basket, desperate attempts to repair a shattered spine. In search of a remedy, I traversed from one doctor to another, one pain clinic to the next, and all I had to do was present my grim x-rays, lay bare my medical chart, and like clockwork, they'd prescribe more opiates to quell my agony.

As the years dragged on, my therapy had brought me no closer to freedom, to the ability to walk once more. Disenchanted with my circumstance, I turned to self-medication, using the opiates to numb the emotional turmoil that gnawed at my soul. It wasn't the physical pain that drove me to this precipice—it was the bitter realization that despite giving my all, I remained trapped in this confining chair.

Each day, my regiment of pills was relentless—a cruel symphony of Oxycontin 80 in the morning, accompanied by five Roxycontin, an orchestra of numbness. I'd push my broken body through therapy, teetering on the edge of endurance, only to numb myself again with another OxyContin 80 and five more Roxycontin beside my devoted wife. The cycle persisted, my final dose delivered just before I sought solace in sleep's embrace, a temporary respite from the never-ending pain.

My life, once vibrant and full of promise, had become a fog of medicated existence, a facade that hid the relentless addiction beneath. With every pill swallowed, I wore the finest disguise—an addiction veiled in the guise of a valid excuse for my suffering. Yet, deep within, I yearned for the strength to break free from the prison of my own making, to reclaim my life from the clutches of addiction and rediscover the light that had long eluded me.

Amidst the wreckage of my shattered spine, I bore the weight of titanium rods, screws, baskets, and plates, visible on those haunting x-rays as a testament to my unyielding pain. Unlike the stories of mere pinched nerves and bulging discs, my excuse was unparalleled—I was paralyzed, a truth no one could refute. It became my leverage, justifying my insatiable addiction to those around me: my family, doctors, therapists, and friends, all unwittingly complicit in my downward spiral.

One fateful day, as my wife picked me up from therapy, my precious daughter accompanied her in the car. Her young voice pierced the fog of my medicated haze, inquiring about the pills that her father consumed religiously. "Mom, what are all those pills that dad takes? Are they really going to kill him?" Her words reverberated through my soul, shattering the illusions I had woven to conceal my secret suffering. My family knew, they knew I was a prisoner to these pills. My desperation drove me to invade the sacred spaces of my loved ones, scavenging their medicine cabinets like a thief in search of the next fix. The consequences were swift, and one by one, I was cast out from their sanctuaries, my shame driving a wedge between us.

Only another addict could understand the consuming anxiety of running out, of taking too much, and the desperation that grips you when the claws of withdrawal sink in. I attempted to quit countless times, only to be ensnared time and again in the siren's call of the drugs that held me captive.

The self-loathing, the rage, the anguish—it was a torment only another addict could comprehend. I found myself shackled to something I could not control, a force that dictated my every move. I was willing to do anything for these pills, to lie, cheat, and steal, betraying the very essence of my soul.

I had never intended to tread this treacherous path, yet here I stood—an addict, ensnared in the clutches of a demon I once believed I could control.

But that moment in the car with my daughter was a turning point, a flash of clarity amid the haze. I knew I couldn't live like this any longer. My trembling hand dialed the number of my doctor, my voice a whisper amidst the cacophony of emotions that raged within me. Even in my medicated stupor, I mustered the courage to confess my years of deceit, my futile attempts to quit, and my dark secret—that I used the opiates to numb the emotional torment more than the physical agony.

With determination, I declared my decision to be done with the pills forever. I sought a clean break from this prison of addiction. But my doctor, calm and resolute, delivered the grim reality of my predicament—I was entangled in a staggering 390 mg of opiates each day. The withdrawal would be unbearable, and he suggested Suboxone or methadone as a lifeline to ease my suffering.

Those words ignited a spark of defiance within me. I was no heroin addict; I would not swap one vice for another. My resolve surged, and I boldly proclaimed that I would go cold turkey, forsaking the crutch that had crippled me for so long.

But amidst my newfound determination, a chilling realization pierced my heart—I had made that life-altering decision while high, a decision that would test my will and resilience like never before. The darkness loomed, but I knew deep down that it was a pivotal step towards reclaiming my life, even if it meant traversing the treacherous road of withdrawal with every ounce of strength I could muster.

Amidst the tumultuous storm of withdrawal, my family rallied around me, becoming unwavering pillars of support. My father, taking a leave of absence from work, and my brother, traveling from California, stood by my side with unwavering determination, ready to help me break free from the clutches of addiction.

In the initial, agonizing days of withdrawal, I plummeted into a torturous nightmare. The remnants of opiates in my body caused relentless days and sleepless nights, marked by shaking, heightened irritability, and an overwhelming stench as the toxins exited. My body rebelled fiercely against the sudden drug deprivation, causing violent vomiting and diarrhea. By the third day, my shower floor was a mess, and my wife remained beside me, despite the anguish I hurled at her.

My grip on reality wavered, with anger and self-inflicted pain being my coping mechanisms. Tortured by insomniac hallucinations of bugs beneath my skin, I was trapped in my deteriorating mental state. In a plea for relief, my family summoned my doctor, whose visit, instead of bringing the anticipated medication, brought a confrontation about my addiction. His blunt declaration, "Matt, you're acting like an addict," served as a sobering mirror. It marked a turning point, awakening a resolve within me. Amidst the ordeal, a newfound hope arose, hinting at a future free from the shackles of addiction.

In the depths of my withdrawals, my doctor offered me a lifeline—a drug called Seroquel, an antipsychotic meant to bring me the elusive gift of sleep. With desperation clawing at my every fiber, I clung to that tiny glimmer of hope, eager to embrace the rest I so desperately craved. As my doctor stepped out to speak with my family, I seized the opportunity and swallowed every Seroquel he had given me, oblivious to the grave danger I was courting.

After a rapid overdose, I was on the verge of a catastrophic health crisis. Though the fear of death wasn't my primary concern, the dread of enduring another day in agonizing withdrawal was. After seven harrowing days, the opiates finally left my system, leading me to vow never to return to them. Throughout this ordeal, my 12-year-old daughter documented her observations and emotions, capturing her confusion, concern, and longing for her father's well-being in a heartfelt journal.

"Day one: my dad is going off all of his pills forever. Dig in, dig deep, and get it done! With a big smiley face."

"Day two: my dad is mean! He says mean things to my mom and to my grandpa. This is all over pills. I don't understand."

"Day three: my dad is as sick as a dog. He's on the shower floor, unable to sit up or talk. He is so sick. I am so worried."

"Day four: (the day of my Seroquel overdose) her journal entry reads this: today is the first day that I saw my grandpa cry. I want someone to give my dad back all of his pills so he can be normal again. MY DAD SCARES ME.!"

Reading my daughter's words deeply affected me, making me realize the pain my addiction caused her. My addiction hadn't only tormented me but also overshadowed my loved ones. Her journal brought me to tears, solidifying my resolve to overcome my addiction and become a father deserving of her love and trust again. The path to healing and redemption wouldn't be easy, but for her sake, my own, and our future, I was committed to escaping the dark grip of opiates and becoming the protective figure she once knew.

For eight years, I fought the battle of recovery with unwavering resolve. Though the allure of opiates still lingered in the recesses of my mind, I had found healthier ways to cope with pain and neuropathy. My relationships had mended, and I was basking in the clarity of sobriety. Life seemed to have turned a new leaf, until fate dealt a devastating blow.

In a heart-stopping moment, a drunk driver collided with my car on the interstate. The devastation was immediate, trapping me with spinal fractures and renewed paralysis. Flashbacks of the past emerged when Dilaudid was given to ease my pain, resembling the return of a familiar, treacherous foe. Addiction's grip tightened, ensnaring me again.

Faced with this dire reality, I came to a profound acceptance. I accepted my fate to the disease of addiction that plagued me and realized that surrendering to a higher power, to God, was my path forward. The shadow of doubt and fear loomed, making me question if I could bear the torment of withdrawal once more. But I sought solace in my spiritual connection and family, asking for support to navigate the darkest chapter of my life. With their unwavering belief in my resolve to break the chains of addiction, we embarked on this daunting recovery journey together.

For more than a year, united, we combated the relentless demon of addiction. I surrendered control over the pain medication, understanding its dominance over me. With my family's vigilance and my steadfast resolve, I gradually reclaimed my life.

Today, on this July day of 2023, I stand with pride, celebrating 10 months of sobriety for the second time in my life. The battle is far from over, and I acknowledge that pain medication will forever be a formidable adversary. But I am no longer afraid. My daily strength comes from my connection with God and a loving family that knows my struggles, knows my aspirations, and will not allow me to falter.

I have learned that recovery is not a solitary journey—it is a collective effort, with the strength of my loved ones and a higher power, bolstering my resolve. My advice to all who read my story is simple: Turn to your creator in your greatest time of need. He will be there for you to hold you in his loving embrace. involve others in your recovery. Surround yourself with those who offer you the best chance for success and commit to the hard work that lies ahead.

Shed the shackles of negativity, both from others and from within. Embrace the belief that your best is enough, and each day, strive to be a better version of yourself. In the beginning, focus on getting through each second, knowing that seconds turn to minutes, minutes to hours, and eventually, days to weeks, weeks to months, and months to years. It does get easier, and life becomes brighter on the other side.

Dig in, dig deep, and get it done. Embrace the power of community, the strength of love, and the unyielding spirit within you. Together, we can conquer the monsters that seek to devour our lives, emerging triumphant, free, and stronger than ever before.

DESPERATION OF A DYING MAN